21st Century Media and Female Mental Health

Fredrika Thelandersson

21st Century Media and Female Mental Health

Profitable Vulnerability and Sad Girl Culture

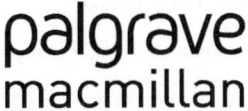

Fredrika Thelandersson
Media and Communication Studies
Lund University
Lund, Sweden

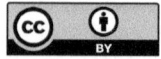

ISBN 978-3-031-16755-3   ISBN 978-3-031-16756-0   (eBook)
https://doi.org/10.1007/978-3-031-16756-0

Cover credit: Iana Sereda / EyeEm/Getty Images

This Palgrave Macmillan imprint is published by the registered company Springer Nature Switzerland AG.
The registered company address is: Gewerbestrasse 11, 6330 Cham, Switzerland

To all the sad girls out there –
You will make it through

ACKNOWLEDGMENTS

This book started out as my doctoral dissertation, which I wrote as a graduate student in media studies at Rutgers University's School of Communication and Information. In the process of turning the text into a book manuscript, I have teased out the main arguments that at the dissertation stage were only subtly expressed. This has involved developing the claims about the double nature of twenty-first-century mental health awareness, which takes shape as both profitable vulnerability and sad girl culture. I have also added a background chapter that traces the history of sad and mad women in the Anglo-American West, which historicizes my understanding of contemporary conceptions of gendered mental illness.

The person that most influenced the early stages of this research project was my doctoral advisor, Jack Bratich, and I thank him for his intellectual generosity and belief in my scholarship. Without his support and guidance this book would not be here today. My dissertation committee members, Marija Dalbello, Mary Chayko, and Rosalind Gill, offered the project encouragement and perspective. Marija was an encouraging and challenging mentor from my first year in the PhD program; without her classes and direction my scholarship would not be where it is today. Thanks to Mary for her insights given to the project and for being an inspirational and educational supervisor to my teaching efforts. And I am so grateful for the support of Ros, whose work has inspired my analytical thinking tremendously—it is an academic rarity and privilege to get firsthand input from the person you singlehandedly cite the most.

Thanks also to the many other people who made my time at Rutgers so enriching and influenced the direction of my work. Susan Keith, thank you for your mentorship as a teacher, colleague, and departmental chair. The community of doctoral students and candidates was a source of inspiration and comfort. Thank you especially to Katie McCollough, Vyshali Manivannan, Henry Boachi, and Omar Hammad.

Thanks to Greg Seigworth and the team behind *Capacious: Journal for Emerging Affect Inquiry* for arranging the inspiring affect conferences in 2015, 2018, and 2019, and for publishing my article about Tumblr sad girls. This book grew out of that first paper I presented at the 2015 conference and was then given significant improvement in the generous peer-review process during the spring of 2017. Parts of Chap. 5 are based on the article I published in *Capacious*, and I hope this book will live as vivid a life as that publication has. The two conferences and the summer school have given me so much intellectual inspiration and an international scholarly home in the most capacious way. I am also thankful to Greg for his feedback and encouragement when this book was only at the proposal stage.

I am so grateful to the American Association of University Women (AAUW) for awarding me with the 2019–2020 American Dissertation Fellowship, without which I would have not been able to focus full time on the dissertation during that last year of writing. It was a remarkable gift to be able to turn my primary attention to research during an entire year, and that dedication definitely made it a better project and book in the end.

Since I left Rutgers, I have gained a new scholarly home in the Department of Communication and Media at Lund University, and the conversations I have had with my wonderful colleagues there have influenced the final form that this manuscript has taken. Thanks especially to my mentor and colleague Helena Sandberg, who is ever-encouraging and inspiring.

Beyond the academy I want to thank Malmö-based leftist organization Krakel, which has given me a non-institutional intellectual home where ideas have flourished. I am especially grateful for the study circle "Psyket i kapitalismen," led by Mirjam Katzin during the fall of 2021. The conversations we had in that forum helped my thinking about psychic life in contemporary capitalism tremendously, and they have most definitely influenced the development of my arguments in this book.

I also want to thank Linda Forsell and the performing arts company PotatoPotato, with whom I shared my research on sad girls, which then resulted in the theater performance SADLAND. It was so inspiring to see my research expressed in new and provocative ways. This experience convinced me of the importance of reaching beyond academic venues to communicate our work to those who are directly affected by it.

Thank you to my family, spread out in Sweden and Germany, who have supported me in every step of the way. And thanks to my nonacademic friends on both sides of the Atlantic for being there, for trying to understand, and for providing support. Ira Potashner, thank you for your continued guidance and professional insights.

Lastly, thank you to the sad girls of Tumblr and Instagram: you have taught and helped me so much. This book is for you.

Contents

Contents

LIST OF FIGURES

CHAPTER 1

Introduction

Sadness and mental health awareness seem to be everywhere in the popular media landscape of the 2020s. From the music streaming service Spotify's wide range of playlists tailored for sad moods (with titles like "Sad Bops," "Down in the Dumps," and "All the feels"), the US premium cable channel HBO adding mental health disclaimers to shows that depict particular ailments, British royal Prince Harry participating in the launch of a mental health app to aid military service members while his wife Meghan Markle revealed that she had been suicidal in their widely publicized interview with Oprah, to one of the biggest pop stars of the moment being Billie Eilish, a young woman making sad, dark songs while openly talking about her own struggles with depression.[1]

The presence of sadness and mental illness awareness in mainstream public culture is a fairly recent phenomenon. Several scholars have defined the media landscape of the early twenty-first century as focused on happiness, creating a culture that privileges the positive and energetic while dismissing pain, injury, and failure.[2] As recently as 2017, pop star Selena Gomez explained her choice to be open about her struggles with anxiety and depression by saying: "We girls, we're taught to be almost too resilient, to be strong and sexy and cool and laid-back … We also need to feel allowed to fall apart."[3] The indirect proposition here was that it was out of the ordinary to speak about such issues in public, and that the general expectation of young women is that they show strength and flexibility at all costs. Along with Gomez's statement, the last decade has seen an increase in representations and conversations about mental health in

© The Author(s) 2023
F. Thelandersson, *21st Century Media and Female Mental Health*,
https://doi.org/10.1007/978-3-031-16756-0_1

popular culture at large. Popular magazines and digital publications are regularly covering issues like depression and anxiety. Countless listicles of celebrities that have opened up about their struggles with mental illness have appeared.[4] Scripted characters with various psychic ailments pop up across the TV and movie landscape.[5] On social media platforms young people are self-identifying with the moniker "sad girl," inhabiting a position that places negative feelings at the forefront. And there is an endless stream of accounts that offer support for various diagnoses and general self-care, made up of both amateurs and mental health professionals who supply their followers with advice and relief.[6]

How did the positive media landscape of the early 2000s turn into one that frequently addresses mental illness and trauma? *21st Century Media and Female Mental Health: Profitable Vulnerability and Sad Girl Culture* charts the shift in Western media culture from a primarily positive and upbeat affective register to one that has space for some talk of negative and downtrodden feelings. I examine the increased visibility of mental illness and sadness in popular Anglo-American media by analyzing a set of texts about depression, anxiety and general mental illness. These texts come from three primary sites—women's magazines, female celebrities, and social media—chosen for their function as purveyors of scripts for how we come to think about and experience mental health and illness.

FRAMEWORK

Drawing on the work of Rosalind Gill, Christina Scharff, Diane Negra, Yvonne Tasker, and others, I situate the increased visibility of mental illness against a backdrop of a neoliberal and postfeminist culture that privileges individualism and personal choice, placing the responsibility for happiness and wellbeing solely on the individual.[7] I look at these contemporary iterations of mental illness specifically in relation to gender, following thinkers who define women as ideal neoliberal subjects.[8] Women in particular are hailed as subjects of capacity that have the potential for great success if they just work hard enough on themselves (more on that below). Depression, however, is associated with debility and the incapacity to act.

Feminist scholars have also written about the psychic life of neoliberalism and postfeminism, paying attention to how contemporary media culture focuses increasingly on the psychological, calling on subjects to work on not only their bodies and careers but also on their moods and attitudes.[9] The feelings that are privileged here tend to be positive ones:

confidence, empowerment, shamelessness, and resilience.[10] Attention has also been given to the appearance of negative affects in this otherwise positive emotional landscape. Examples of this include Amy Shields Dobson and Akane Kanai's study of affective dissonances in post-recessional television shows aimed at young women, Shani Orgad and Gill's exploration of mediated female rage in the #MeToo era, and Helen Wood's examination of the prevalence of the word "fuck" in contemporary feminist speech.[11] These analyses present a complicated affective landscape. The presence of affective dissonances may be read as a problematization of the "accessibility and appeal of highly individualist career-oriented lifestyles idealised in cultural mythologies of powerful "can-do" girls."[12] But in other instances female rage enters the mediated public sphere only to be "simultaneously contained and disavowed."[13] And in yet another figuration, the repeated use of "fuck" might signal an irreverent feminist rage that rejects respectability politics along the lines of gender, race, class, and sexuality, in an ultimately hopeful way.[14] Rage in particular appeared as a powerful affect from which to build feminist politics after the 2016 election of Donald Trump.[15] Activist-scholar Brittney Cooper has, in the tradition of Audre Lorde, called for an "eloquent rage" that is especially important for black feminist action as a source of energy that gives strength to keep fighting as well as clarity in what needs to be changed.[16]

Orgad and Gill have brilliantly described how the imperative to confidence for women within twenty-first-century media culture often works to dismantle feminist messages of their structural critique and place the solution to social injustice on the individual.[17] By working on their confidence and self-esteem, women are presumed to overcome systemic issues. Orgad and Gill also acknowledge a seemingly contradictory move, which they call "the vulnerability turn," where women are encouraged to express their weaknesses, insecurities and self-doubts.[18] But rather than challenge the confidence cult, this vulnerability works to reinforce it, where brands often introduce insecurity only to replace it with "defiant individualism."[19]

Angela McRobbie also identifies this tendency to allow weakness in contemporary media culture, but she defines it as the "imperfect" and places it within a triangulation of affects expressed as the "perfect—imperfect—resilience."[20] Here the perfect encourages women to succeed meritocratically in a highly competitive environment that favors a neoliberal "leadership-feminism." The imperfect is then expressed as a response to the "unviability of the emphasis on success," but it is articulated within severely limited parameters and quickly followed by a resilience that "springs into existence as a 'bounce-back' mechanism."[21]

My book takes off from these previous theoretizations and looks at what I call the "turn to sadness" in twenty-first-century media culture. My analysis shares similarities with both Orgad and Gill's vulnerability turn and McRobbie's imperfect, in that it describes what I term a "profitable vulnerability" that allows for market-friendly iterations of weakness that fit within the otherwise largely positive affective register of mainstream media culture. But in addition to this profitable vulnerability, I also delineate more spacious ways of feeling bad within the sad girl culture(s) of social media. What I hope to do in this analysis is to look closer at how sadness as both diagnosis and general affect is allowed to take up space in various media texts and what it can tell us about the state of psychic ailments, healing, and recovery in relation to neoliberal capitalist knowledge systems.

The Sites of Study

Women's magazines have long functioned as guides for women and girls that model how to live life in the most ideal or proper way. McRobbie writes in her classic study of the girls' magazine *Jackie* that publications in this genre "define and shape the woman's world, spanning every stage from early childhood to old age [where] the exact nature of the woman's role is spelt out in detail, according to her age and status."[22] One aspect of this guidance was the supportive function provided by these magazines, where experts answered questions about everything from relationships to medical problems.

For a long time, women's magazines were a stable fixture of the media landscape, with various outlets aimed at specific niche segments of the female audience (like working mothers, sophisticated black women, fashion-forward twenty-somethings, and so on). Since the start of the twenty-first century and the rise of digital media, however, women's magazines have struggled with declining revenues as advertisers and readers move to free online platforms.[23] The traditional magazines still hold the role of advice givers but celebrities, influencers, and peer networks on social media have also stepped into that role and now function as similar guiding lights. *21st Century Media and Female Mental Health* thus looks at three sites——magazines, celebrities, and social media networks——to understand the contemporary discourse around gendered mental health. I understand these various media sites as actively defining what it means to suffer from depression and anxiety, as well as providing solutions for how to deal with these ailments.

When it comes to social media, the popularity of various platforms and the trends that proliferate on them shift with great speed. I do not make any claims to definite truths about the culture of various social media platforms, rather I hope to provide a snapshot of what the conversations around mental health looked like during the 2010s on the specific platforms discussed. And as any astute observer of social media knows, niche cultures proliferate with remarkable speed and no static description of them can accurately portray their complex dynamics. Nevertheless, I here attempt to capture a glimpse of how mental illness and sadness took shape in the digital worlds of the 2010s.

Within the frames of this book I define the contemporary moment as the period from 2008 and onward, with an understanding that the cultural and social landscape in the West was significantly affected by the 2008 financial crisis and the subsequent bank bailouts and austerity measures. The financial recession can be read as the starting point for the current precarious state of life in the West. The data collection for this project originally covered the time frame 2008-2018, as a way to make it manageable. The bulk of material that my analysis is based on comes from this period, but relevant events that took place after this time frame has also been included where appropriate. The COVID-19 pandemic, for example, started after I had concluded my first analysis of the material. This is thus not a study of how COVID has changed how mental health is talked about in the media. It is rather an examination of how the popular media landscape has, successively since 2008, become more and more intimate and conducive for conversations around previously private topics like depression and anxiety, something that came to a head during the pandemic year of 2020. Because what became obvious early on in the COVID-19 crisis was the extent to which the media we consume in our everyday life function not only as information suppliers, but also very much as nodes of support in uncertain times. As people all over the world were stuck inside, many turned to friends as well as celebrities on social media to stay connected and get support. The study of how various media shape our understanding of mental health is in this sense of heightened relevance as the world encounters the new normal of a post-COVID-19 world.

Guiding Questions

21ˢᵗ Century Media and Female Mental Health examines the contemporary structure of feeling that produces these increased representations of mental illness.[24] I ask how female subjects are hailed as mentally ill in various mediated spaces. My analysis is focused on depression and anxiety, as terms referring both to medicalized discourses of control and psychosocial affects like vulnerability, sadness, and melancholia. Other common diagnoses, such as bipolar disorder, also appeared repeatedly in my media archive and have also been included.

My analysis adds to the understanding of the changing media landscape of advice-giving, from magazines to celebrities and peers on social media. It contributes to the field of feminist media studies by studying the entanglement of emotions and popular feminism.

The key questions guiding me fall into two categories, first a set of questions concerning the gendered effects of neoliberalism regarding health:

> What do the contemporary conversations around mental health look like in feminine/female dominated media spaces? What definitions and solutions are provided? And how do the discourses around these sad affects relate to an otherwise upbeat and positive media culture? What does it mean that a culture that tends to privilege the positive now is making way for talk of mental illnesses like depression and anxiety? Are we seeing a repudiation of the "happiness industry" or is it merely another side of the same coin? What happens with the infinitely capable neoliberal subject when she acknowledges weakness?

And a second set of questions referring to the role of digital media platforms in these processes:

> What meanings and connections emerge in digital spaces when women share their experiences of mental illness with each other there? Do the definitions shared contribute new and more spacious ways of feeling bad? And what potential for change in perceptions around mental illness do these discourses provide?

These questions take a critical approach to media culture by interrogating how meanings are produced around issues of mental health. But I am also following scholars like Sarah Projansky, who "draws on a feminist media studies methodology in pursuit of optimistic anti-racist queer readings" of representations of girlhood.[25] In my research I have looked for potentially subversive aspects in portrayals of depression and anxiety. Here I have also taken into account the often-unequal representation of who suffers from mental illness. A certain kind of girl sadness is often associated with white and thin bodies[26] and the expressions of sadness and pain that received the most attention online during the time period I examine have been criticized for only referring to white women.[27] But the online discourse around mental health also includes conversations that question exclusionary representations of what it means to suffer psychically. Examples include artist and mental health advocate Dior Vargas' "People of Color and Mental Illness Photo Project" which was started in 2014 to raise awareness about mental health in communities of color and Sad Girls Club, an Instagram account and in person meetup group that focuses specially on the experience of women of color living with mental illness.[28] *Teen Vogue* also publishes pieces about the connection between mental health and structural inequalities regularly.[29]

It is particularly within the online spaces that I have found what resembles subversive portrayals of living with depression, anxiety, and other diagnoses. I discuss the activity by some of the sad girls on Tumblr and Instagram with the scholarly activist collective *Institute for Precarious Consciousness*'s notion of a "precarity-focused consciousness raising" to move out from under the debilitating grip of anxiety, which they define as the dominant affect of the contemporary moment.[30]

One of the indirect questions for this project has also been whether or not the mere presence of mental health awareness constitutes a challenge to a culture focused on happiness and success. In other words, is it automatically a "good" thing to talk more about depression, anxiety, and other issues that affect our psyches? The short answer is "it's complicated." The example of Meghan Markle revealing that she had been suicidal while living as a royal in a widely publicized interview with Oprah is illustrative in this regard. On the one hand, a cynical reading of the situation might be that Markle and her prince husband choose to align themselves with mental health causes and revealed some personal struggle to appear authentic and relatable (a belief expressed by various pundits at the time). This analysis can be true but one must at the same time acknowledge that Markle's confession opened up space for the acknowledgement of what it means to live with depression and suicidal thoughts in social contexts where such issues have been taboo.[31] Such is the complexity of mental health awareness – it is rarely an easy either or of "good" versus "bad" awareness, but instead a nuanced web of elements that conform to existing power structures.

My aim with this book is to explore multiple aspects of contemporary gendered mental health discourse, both the "bad" and the "good." The arguments of Orgad and Gill and McRobbie mentioned above, which describe the presence of vulnerability and weakness in media culture as largely feeding back into the neoliberal logic of confidence and resilience, are compelling.[32] I follow their understandings and add primarily two elements: 1) I look at what the sanctioned vulnerability looks like——how it functions as a generator of authenticity that forms close relations between brand and follower; and 2) I do a reparative reading that also acknowledges the more spacious ways of feeling bad that the increased conversations around mental health open up, primarily on social media within the sad girl culture there. I hope the reader can keep these two aspects in mind at the same time and hold space for complexity and nuance.

Notes on Methodology

In terms of methodology, I conduct a feminist media studies analysis of discourses around mental health in popular culture and on social media, using a multi-methods approach that moves across magazines, celebrities, social media. I employ content and textual analysis of magazines and celebrity performances, and an online ethnography of multiple iterations of the Internet phenomenon of the sad girl.

As mentioned above, the project focuses on three main sites—articles about mental health and illness in two publications aimed at women and girls (*Cosmopolitan* and *Teen Vogue*); female celebrities who have spoken publicly about dealing with depression and anxiety (primarily Demi Lovato[33] and Selena Gomez); and socially mediated expressions of depression, anxiety, and general sadness online (sad girls on Tumblr and Instagram, as well as the specific cases of Audrey Wollen, Sad Girls Y Qué, Sad Girls Club, and My Therapist Says). In my analysis, I have looked for specific mentions of depression, anxiety, and diagnoses like bipolar disorder, while also taking note of statements that convey related psychosocial affects like vulnerability, sadness, and melancholia without directly naming diagnoses. I have asked questions about the way in which depression and anxiety are talked about; who gets to speak about it; what the solutions and responses presented are; and how these conversations relate to power/ knowledge structures, whether directly or implicitly.

In addition to Projansky's "optimistic anti-racist queer readings" of representations of girlhood I also work with Eve Kosofsky Sedgwick's calls for reparative, rather than paranoid, critical reading.[34] For Sedgwick, critical theory has for too long been invested in a "hermeneutics of suspicion" which analyzes the world in a paranoid way that always aims to uncover a negative or damaging truth.[35] The problem with paranoid reading is that it presumes sinister intentions behind the surface and that it places ultimate faith in what exposing those intentions might do for the greater good. Sedgwick proposes instead an understanding of paranoia as "one kind of epistemological practice among other, alternative ones," and urges scholars to also engage in reparative readings.[36] A reparative position involves a "seeking of pleasure" and an openness to optimistic readings of a text or situation.[37] In relation to contemporary mental health discourses, this means looking for potentially subversive or reparative aspects in portrayals of depression, anxiety, and other mental illness.

THE EMERGENCE OF TWENTY-FIRST-CENTURY SADNESS

Women's affective states have a long history of being pathologized under names like neurasthenia, hysteria, and schizophrenia.[38] In culture, the sad and mad woman has appeared as various popular figures: the Victorian madwoman, the hysteric, the schizophrenic, and the Prozac-consuming American woman of the 1990s, to name a few. In Chap. 2 I trace the lineage of these figures since the early modern period up until today.

Historically, women's sad experiences have been classified as pathologies leading to institutionalization and confinement. In the contemporary moment, they tend to be medicalized within a biochemical discourse that reverts to (deinstitutionalized) psychotropic drugs and psychotherapy as solutions. In this way, the current pathologization of women's sad experiences takes place within a neoliberal framework that does not position them as abject and (completely) other, but instead renders them intelligible within a larger culture of self-help in which the individual is responsible for her own wellbeing.[39] In this framework, all ties between health and structures of inequality are severed, and any attempts at politicizing widespread ill health are thwarted. *21ˢᵗ Century Media and Female Mental Health* shows that this mode of thinking about mental health is dominant, but not all-encompassing in contemporary popular culture. There are plenty of examples of a profitable vulnerability that is shared to strengthen brands' authenticity, but there are also several sites where ties between mental wellbeing and larger power structures are being made, most explicitly in *Teen Vogue* and among the sad girls on Instagram.

One of the arguments I make in this book is that the figure of the sad girl emerged as an indirect response to a media culture that required women in particular to be strong, empowered, and confident. The first example of this is the artist Lana del Rey and the splash she made when she debuted with a homemade video for the song "Video Games" in late 2011. The video went viral and she became famous overnight, and when her debut album *Born to Die* was released in January 2012 it topped the charts in eleven countries. But alongside the hype and popularity came an onslaught of criticism and vitriol from both Internet users and mainstream media outlets like the *New York Times*.[40] The music video for the song "Video Games" is a mash-up of 1950s Hollywood aesthetics, boys on skateboards, a drunk and stumbling woman being helped to a car, palm trees, the iconic L.A. hotel Chateau Marmont and del Rey herself looking sultry with plump lips and her hair made up in a 1960s beehive.[41] The song is ostensibly about a girl very much in love with a boy who likes to play video games, and who gives her all to be with him, with the chorus going "It's you, it's you, it's all for you / Everything I do / I tell you all the time / Heaven is a place on Earth with you." The song and video, together with the following single "Born to Die" and the album with the same title, emphasized submissiveness and a tendency towards self-destructive behavior. These sentiments stood in stark contrast to the refrain of self-empowerment that dominated pop at the time.[42] One music journalist described it as follows:

> Nowhere else in mass culture have young people, especially women, been allowed to feel so unvexed about their desires, even if those desires are constrained to the relatively superficial, glitter-sprayed longings of a Ke$ha rager: 'We're taking control/We've got what we want/We do what you don't.'[43]

The problem with del Rey, argued the same journalist, is that she "sings as a woman who doesn't know what she wants," which was why she appeared as a provocation to some. NPR's music critic Ann Powers argued that del Rey's "persona relies on classic femme fatale allure, but without the usual "girl power" update … So women find her troubling; she embodies the worst part of being a girl."[44] In the pop cultural climate of the time, del Rey's passivity and sadness was upsetting in its turn away from (post)feminist can-do spirit. Media studies scholar Catherine Vigier provided the following analysis at the time:

> One of the problems is that, after a decade in which women were told that they had everything it took to get ahead, and that the playing-field was somehow level in our new, post-feminist world, it was disturbing to many to see a woman recast herself as an old-fashioned male fantasy and to seemingly embrace submissiveness, and to dress as if she were nostalgic for the days before women's liberation.[45]

For Vigier, one of the main draws of del Rey was that she spoke for the women who felt left out of the empowerment feminism of the day and gave "expression to some of the profound dissatisfactions that women continue to feel."[46] This interpretation is similar to what artist Audrey Wollen expressed a few years later when she proposed a "Sad Girl Theory" to reconceptualize female sadness as a form of protest through images posted on her Instagram account.[47] For Wollen, women sharing photographs of themselves crying or otherwise publicly displaying their sadness should not be seen as expressions of weakness, but should instead be interpreted as modes of dissent in a patriarchal world that requires women to smile.

This is not to say that del Rey and Wollen were the inventors or originators of this kind of sad expression, rather they exist in the long lineage of sad women (explored in Chap. 2). But they are examples of a kind of sad aesthetic that emerged in the 2010s and very much also took shape online. Zoe Alderton, who writes about the contemporary aesthetics of self-harm, describes it as "a newer kind of 'Sad' Aesthetic [that] has come exclusively from the internet generation and new modes of mass communication."[48] She locates this aesthetic as especially connected to the social media platform Tumblr and the "Tumblr Teen Girl Aesthetic" which is "both powerfully emotive and deeply ironic."[49] Important to note here is that the girls associated with this kind of sad expression tend to be white and thin, and the possibilities this position offer are thus limited (something I explore more in Chap. 5).[50]

21ˢᵗ Century Media and Female Mental Health explores how this sad aesthetic has spread from the lesser-known corners of the internet and into popular culture at large. In addition to a higher presence of sad songs among the top charts,[51] my research shows that there was an increase in magazine coverage of depression/anxiety and celebrity confessions of living with mental illness from 2015 and onwards. I am not arguing that there was a straight line of causation or influence from Internet subculture to the mainstream, rather I want to call attention to a general turn to sadness on multiple levels of popular culture.

This new visibility surrounding issues of mental illness takes multiple forms. On the one hand there is an awareness of diagnoses and different conditions in ways that seek to normalize issues as common and "just like any other disease." Discourses in this vein largely try to present depression and anxiety in easily digestible and nonthreatening ways, following Akane Kanai's work on "affectively relatable" online selves that touch upon difficult subjects but do so with self-deprecating humor that serves to defuse the seriousness of the problems.[52] These representations are found largely in *Cosmopolitan's* coverage of mental illness, among celebrities and microcelebrities, and in some of the more commercial "sad girl" accounts on social media. This kind of representation of mental illness largely takes the shape of a "profitable vulnerability" that serves to show acceptance and tolerance of weakness while keeping a distance/remaining unthreatening. This vulnerability becomes profitable in that it strengthens the authenticity of a brand, something seen clearly in the celebrity health narrative of Demi Lovato (explored in Chap. 4).

Another aspect of the heightened visibility of mental health is the increased intimacy of celebrity and influencer culture. Traditional celebrities are becoming more ordinary and tend to open up more about their personal lives to create and maintain strong connections with fans, while "regular" people turn into microcelebrities by building intense and intimate connections with followers.[53] Disclosing a mental illness diagnosis can be a successful way of building up these bonds and often serves to strengthen brands based on authenticity. At the same time the media outlets that provide advice and where women have traditionally turned to for support, like magazines, largely reach audiences via social media feeds that are also filled with content from celebrities, influencers, and peers. In this way the various media spaces blend into each other and all function as nodes of support.

But alongside examples of profitable vulnerability are also more critical accounts where mental wellbeing is presented as a more complex issue and frequently connected to power structures and inequality. These accounts are largely found in *Teen Vogue*, whose contemporary branding attempts to construct girls and young women as political subjects with agency, and among the more radical sad girls on Instagram who tend to critique the US mental health care system and the state of capitalism.[54] This kind of sad girl culture offers more spacious ways of feeling bad that include both a systemic critique and direct support.

ON TERMINOLOGY, CONTEXTUAL SPECIFICATIONS, AND INTERSECTIONALITY

A note on terminology and the contextual specifications of the book is appropriate here. First, I largely use mental health and mental illness interchangeably throughout the book. This is partly due to a linguistic choice, repeating "mental illness" over and over would become tedious. But it is also a reflection of the discourses I analyze, where the two terms are used interchangeably to designate both "heathy" and "ill" aspects of the psyche. Mental health awareness generally encompasses factors that are both "good" and "bad" for a healthy mind, whereas mental illness awareness tends to mean knowledge about specific diagnoses. There is a slippage here, then, but it is largely influenced by a slippage present in the popular discourses examined, where definitions of what is exactly entailed by "depression" and "anxiety" are often absent. This lack of clear definitions is itself an aspect of the popular discourses, and in my analysis I ask about what meanings are actually conveyed about what it means to be "depressed," "anxious," or "bipolar."

Second, this book focuses on media texts from the Anglo-American world, with a primarily US perspective on discourses around mental health and illness. I thus make no claims to account for non-Western debates around these topics, even if a global perspective surely would add interesting insights into how the psyche is conceived of in the contemporary world, such an effort is far beyond the scope of this book.

Additionally, within the US-European context, the emphasis is, when it comes to magazines and celebrities, on mainstream media discourse, which tends to reflect a largely white female demographic. In the world of magazines, the assumed subject addressed by *Cosmopolitan* is a white one in that race is not addressed in a majority of pieces. It looks a bit different in *Teen Vogue*, where racism is a recurring topic and the higher rates of depression among people of color are repeatedly acknowledged. Among celebrities the majority of stars who have spoken out about diagnoses or traumas tend to be white or white-passing. And on social media, the sad girl culture examined is largely made up of white subjects, with a few significant exceptions. These are Sad Girls Y Qué, a Mexican group of young women mobilizing the sad girl figure as a protest against machismo culture, and Sad Girls Club, an Instagram account and meet-up group that explicitly focuses on women of color dealing with mental health issues.

In acknowledging the often-presumed whiteness of the subject addressed in the media texts, I hope to avoid falling into the assumption that depression and the like effects everyone the same and always looks the same. The way mental illness is experienced is highly determined by one's immediate circumstances as well as family and cultural histories. There is a rich body of scholarship on racial melancholia that connects histories of colonialism, slavery, and genocide to the present, and defines "the affective life of racialized existence and the psychic impact of racism as a form of loss and trauma."[55] Saidiya Hartman, for example, describes depression as part of the "afterlife of slavery," alongside "skewed life chances, limited access to health and education, premature death, incarceration, and impoverishment."[56] Similarly, after the 2015 Charleston church massacre, in which a white supremacist terrorist shot nine African Americans attending bible study, Claudia Rankine defined "the condition of black life" as one of mourning.[57] This line of thinking acknowledges the lived experience of belonging to an historically marginalized group, whose life prospects are severely limited by ongoing and historical structural violence. The experience of depression for a black subject in the US might be very different than for a "white and middle- class subject for whom feeling bad is frequently a mystery because it doesn't fit a life in which privilege and comfort make things seem fine on the surface."[58] The narratives of mental illness in the media discourses that this book examines largely belong to the latter category here, where painful feelings are seen as a mystery solved by the logic of biomedical diagnoses. I try to show how even that subject and the pathologizations of her moods and behavior are socioculturally bound up in particular power/knowledge relations (in Chap. 2, I attempt to trace what that has looked like historically). But the focus here then is predominantly on the mainstream conceptions of mental health that, often without making it explicit, assumes a white and otherwise carefree subject.

Neoliberalism, Governmentality, and Biopolitics

It is also appropriate to define some of the core theoretical concepts that underlie my analysis. To start, my understanding of the contemporary cultural, social, and economic moment is informed by critical thinkers who define today's Western society as a neoliberal capitalist society. I adhere to a broad definition of neoliberalism as the "political, economic, and social arrangements within society that emphasize market relations, re-tasking the role of the state, and individual responsibility."[59] The ubiquity of market logics and the accompanying demand of the individual to fend for herself in all stages of life is central to my use of the concept. Neoliberalism reaches beyond economic and social policy and influences the formation of our subjectivities.

I follow scholars who have theorized neoliberalism through the Foucauldian concept of governmentality.[60] Governmentality refers to the activities by which a state governs over its citizens. Importantly, within this framework government is not understood simply as institutions of political and economic policy, rather as "a continuum, which extends from political government right through to forms of self-regulation."[61] Foucault refers to these "forms of self-regulation" as "technologies of the self," which are central to the notion of governmentality.[62] They are essential because they denote the ways in which we come to relate to ourselves and make sense of ourselves, and within Foucault's theoretical framework they are closely linked to systems of governance.

For Thomas Lemke, Foucault's writings and lectures on governmentality aimed "to show how the modern sovereign state and the modern autonomous individual co-determine each other's emergence."[63] That is, to show that the development of subjectivity goes hand in hand with the development of the state. The way we become subjects is inextricably linked to the way the governing body of society exercises its control. So, under a neoliberal system of governance, our subjectivities are structured according to a neoliberal rationale. The extension of market logics into all areas of society extends to the level of individuation, and encourages, or demands, that individuals become entrepreneurial subjects with full responsibility for their own lives.[64] Within this logic, something like poverty is not a circumstance with a negative influence over the individual beyond her control; instead, it is the task of the individual to rise above such a circumstance and on her own create a life worth living.

Biopolitics is another important Foucauldian concept that is closely linked to the idea of governmentality. For Foucault, biopolitics is the management of the life of a population, of monitoring and controlling things like health, birthrate, and longevity of a people.[65] Starting in the eighteenth century, political power stopped being exercised only in the giving or taking of life, and became occupied with the wellbeing of the population. Initially this concern arose from specific problems of illnesses, lack of sanitation in towns, and accidents, but soon the management of life became a way for state and police authorities to control and surveil its subjects. Nikolas Rose writes, "from this moment on, politics would have to address the vital processes of human existence: the size and quality of the population; reproduction and human sexuality; conjugal, parental, and familial relations; health and disease; birth and death."[66] One of the most blatant examples of this exercise of power over life is the practice of eugenics in the first half of the twentieth century, which involved elaborate strategies of reproductive control so as to secure a future "welfare of the nation" based on a belief that some physical characteristics were superior to others.[67] But biopolitics also works in less flagrant ways, and remains integral to the exercise of power in the twenty-first century.

In relation to neoliberalism, biopolitics becomes an important way to think about the continued reach of authorities of power in regulating our lives. What is remarkable with the neoliberal configuration is the visible withdrawal of the state in terms of cuts to welfare programs and deregulation of financial markets, which seem to suggest that there is less governance over our lives. Several thinkers have shown that this is not the case, that we instead are being governed in a "new" way, primarily by means of self-regulation.[68] The state (or whatever form the exercise of power takes) is still invested in managing and controlling the life of the population but has displaced the governing of its citizens from social institutions to the individuals themselves. Today this is seen clearly in the ubiquity of self-tracking and self-monitoring digital technologies like pregnancy apps and devices like fitbits, where users record their own activities, physical sensations, and mood changes. The information collected is automatically shared with the corporation owning the app or digital platform, and frequently also shared to users' social media networks. This has given rise to what scholars like Deborah Lupton call the "quantified self.[69] This self is imbued with an entrepreneurial spirit of constant evaluation and optimization. The neoliberal subject, then, is "an 'enterprising' subject: a calculating, self-reflexive, 'economic' subject; one that calculates about itself and works upon itself in order to better itself."[70]

Wendy Brown states that "neo-liberal subjects are controlled *through* their freedom ... because of neoliberalism's *moralization* of the consequences of this freedom."[71] Similarly, Lupton writes that "people are compelled to make themselves central to their own lives when they take on the ethical project of selfhood."[72] Working on oneself in neoliberal society is not an act of self-indulgence but of virtue. We may be free to do whatever we want but we are morally and ethically obliged to "care" for ourselves not only for our own wellbeing, but for the wellbeing of the greater good.[73]

There is a connection here between the call for self-responsibilization and the expert knowledge that guides these processes of self-work. The various modes of self-governance outlined above are influenced, or directly formed, by certain kinds of professional expertise that are closely tied to governments. The relation between expertise and government is a reciprocal one,[74] where what is considered "good, healthy, normal, virtuous, efficient or profitable" is also an affirmation of the contemporary modes of political governance.[75] Notably, this relation is not one of all-pervasive social control, but rather distributed into sometimes contradictory recommendations for living. Rose and Peter Miller argue that the role of expertise is to enact "assorted attempts at the calculated administration of diverse aspects of conduct through countless, often competing, local tactics of education, persuasion, inducement, management, incitement, motivation and encouragement."[76] This expertise is doled out in official governmental programs as well as various types of "lifestyle media" such as advice-giving in magazines and self-help books.

It is thus within this context of self-optimization and work on the self that twenty-first-century discourses of mental health and illness take shape.

Postfeminism and Popular Feminism

A note on the use of postfeminism and popular feminism is also needed. The scholarly field of feminist media studies, which I am in dialogue with, has employed the term postfeminism to identify the role of feminism in the Western media landscape of the 1990s and the early 2000s. In a much-cited piece from 2007, Gill defined a postfeminist sensibility which permeated media culture at the time. This was signified by a view of femininity as "a bodily property; the shift from objectification to subjectification; an emphasis upon self-surveillance, monitoring and self-discipline; a focus on individualism, choice and empowerment; the dominance of a makeover paradigm; and a resurgence of ideas about natural sexual difference."[77] Gill makes the argument that the qualities privileged and emphasized within a postfeminist sensibility fits remarkably well with the dictates of twenty-first-century neoliberalism, so much so that women are the ideal neoliberal subjects, constantly called upon to work on and improve themselves so as to become good laboring subjects. Since then, Gill and others have further developed the concept of a postfeminist sensibility, adding, as mentioned above, that both postfeminism and neoliberalism emphasize not only bodily transformation but also psychic improvement. Drawing on Judith Butler's notion of the "psychic life of power," Gill and Christina Scharff describe the psychic life of postfeminism and neoliberalism.[78] The notion of "psychic life" designates the central role of power in creating and forming our subjectivities.[79] For Gill and others what marks twenty-first-century media is an intense focus on the psychological and a "psychologization of surveillance."[80] As previously mentioned, there are now calls to not only work on the body but also the psyche, to approve one's self-esteem and confidence. The postfeminist and neoliberal subject has to continually work on not only its entrepreneurial skills, but its *affects*.

The theorization of postfeminism has, during the 2010s, been complicated by the emergence of a very visible popular feminism in Western media culture. The relatively new popularity of feminism does not, however, mean that a postfeminist sensibility is now absent from culture. Nor that the messages aimed at women are now straightforwardly feminist in a politically radical way. The feminism that is seen in mainstream media culture is one that sees visibility as an end goal in itself (naming something as feminist becomes more important than working for actual change in laws or policies) and is largely "brandable [and] commensurate with market logics."[81] In relation to this popular feminism a postfeminist sensibility has taken on a new and more subtle form, where feminism is not completely repudiated but seen as obviously important and rearticulated in "purely individual terms that stress choice, empowerment, and competition."[82] Orgad and Gill's definition of a confidence culture that presents individual women's work on their own confidence as solutions to structural gender inequalities is an apt example of this.

I use the term postfeminist throughout the book to designate this articulation of neoliberal logics in gendered ways, to signify a sensibility that both repudiates feminist notions of structural change and embraces a hollow and individualized feminism.

Feminist Approaches to Affect

Lastly, I want to acknowledge the feminist affect theoretical perspectives that have influenced my own thinking about negative affects like depression and anxiety, as individual, social, and political. Feminist scholars have been interested in the relationships between affect, knowledge, and power for a long time, captured succinctly in the second-wave feminist slogan "the personal is political." Underlying this concern have been attempts to "interrogate the gendered nature of the reason/emotion binary," which "throughout the history of Western thought ... has functioned to exclude women (and other bodies outside the white, masculine mainstream) from 'legitimate' knowledge production."[83] Elevating the emotional has been a way of legitimizing and politicizing experiences/ knowledges that have traditionally been discounted on the grounds of not being "reasonable."

Feminist scholars have also been on the forefront of the "affective turn" in academia, as it has moved away from "the text and discourse as key theoretical touchstones" to recenter the body in scholarly/intellectual thought.[84] Scholars like Sara Ahmed, Lauren Berlant, Ann Cvetkovich, Sianne Ngai, and Sedgwick have stressed that affects have a place in the public sphere, and that the public is likewise present in our emotional lives.[85] Importantly, these thinkers do not advocate privileging the personal over the public. Cvetkovich, for example, has argued that traditional feminist theory has overemphasized the ability of personal and communal healing practices to function as solutions to complex social and collective problems.[86] Feminist approaches within the affect theoretical framework have instead analyzed the "complex imbrication" of the emotional and the structural.[87] Ahmed has argued that we look both at the "structure of feeling"[88] and the "feelings of structure," suggesting that "feelings might be how structures get under our skin."[89] Feminist affect theoretical approaches thus offers a way to understand how our inner lives are influenced by power/knowledge structures, and vice versa.

This approach also echoes the influential work of Arlie Russell Hochschild who argued already in 1983 that emotions are managed and disciplined according to particular "feeling rules" in both the public and private (Gill and Kanai use this concept to define the "feeling rules of neoliberalism," which I use as an analytical tool throughout the book).[90] Making a crucial connection to capitalism, she held that emotions could be exploited for profit in the form of "emotional labor." More recently emotions have been linked to the market in Eva Illouz's work on "emotional capitalism."[91] She argues that our economic relations have become increasingly intimate and emotional, while our intimate lives have been restructured in economic terms. Here, feelings are rationalized, measured, and controlled.

Affect theory thus offers crucial perspectives for understanding how our psychic lives are affected by and constituted through our socio-cultural circumstances.

CHAPTER OUTLINE

After the introduction offered in this first chapter, the second chapter traces a brief history of how women's mental health has been pathologized in the American and European West since the start of the modern period. It examines figures of sad and mad women, like the Victorian madwoman, the hysteric, the schizophrenic, and the Prozac-consuming American woman of the 1990s. It traces historical trends in diagnoses, from nineteenth-century neurasthenia and hysteria to twentieth-century schizophrenia and anorexia. Here I also try to account for the historical development of the medical fields of psychology and psychiatry and how they have related to contemporary gender conventions. Alongside this history, I account for feminist interpretations of these various pathologizations. I hope to show that mental illness diagnoses are neither completely discursive (socially and linguistically constructed) nor fixed neurological truths (biological facts of life that always look the same), but emerge and take shape in a complex interplay between sociocultural discourses and an ever-developing medical science.

The third chapter——"Mental Health in Magazines: Relatability and Critique in *Cosmopolitan* and *Teen Vogue*"——looks at how the online editions of these two magazines covered depression, anxiety, and related topics during the time period 2008-2018. It builds on an archive of more than 250 *Cosmopolitan* articles and over 500 *Teen Vogue* pieces to catalogue the differences in style, voice, and representations around depression and mental health in the two outlets. *Cosmopolitan*'s coverage is largely focused on being easygoing and relatable, with much of their coverage taking a distanced and lighthearted approach to issues of mental health. *Teen Vogue* generally takes a more serious approach to issues of mental distress, shown in their adoption of the language of mental health advocacy with frequent mentions of stigma and the importance of speaking out. The differences between the two are highlighted by looking at how the two outlets covered the same celebrity events and study of the antidepressant drug Paxil. I argue that the attitudes towards mental health found in these two publications are representative of larger approaches, where *Cosmo*'s tongue-in-cheek coverage exemplifies a profitable vulnerability that has become firmly established in popular media. *Teen Vogue* on the other hand reflects a critical and morally aware sad girl culture that offers more spacious ways of feeling bad while acknowledging the role of structural inequality in mental health.

The fourth chapter——"Celebrity Mental Health: Intimacy, Ordinariness, and Repeated Self-Transformation"——examines celebrities who have spoken out about their own struggles with mental illness and explored themes of sadness and weakness in their work. The logic at work in celebrity confessions is that when a famous person comes out and reveals that they are suffering they communicate to fans that it is okay to feel that way. The chapter focuses primarily on pop stars Demi Lovato and Selena Gomez as representatives of traditional celebrities being open about their mental health. It also briefly discusses artist Lana del Rey's sad persona and her influence on the music scene. Through these cases, I discuss the increasing ordinariness of celebrities, who now have to maintain the relationship with their fans via myriad social media channels that put excessive focus on intimacy and "realness," a framework within which being open about mental illness becomes an enhancing feature of an "authentic" brand rather than something to be ashamed of.

Lovato's celebrity health narrative shows how mental distress can be successfully folded into a celebrity brand and enhance its market value, as they have been able to make a literal profit off of work that utilizes the tragic events in their life while reinforcing a neoliberal ethos of self-work and self-transformation, exemplifying profitable vulnerability. But this cannot be read only through a cynical lens that highlights the profitable elements of their suffering, because in sharing their story fans who have been through similar things are able to connect with and give support to each other. Gomez's health narrative can be read in a comparable way——she waited to share her struggles until the cultural climate was conducive to framing her problems as something that enhanced rather than detracted from her celebrity brand. But at the same time, in the act of speaking publicly about her issues she also opened up new spaces for talking about things like depression, anxiety, and bipolar disorder. The analysis of these health narratives shows that profitable vulnerability and supportive conversations around mental distress exist in tension with each other in the world of celebrity media.

The fifth chapter——"Social Media Sadness: Sad Girl Culture and Radical Ways of Feeling Bad"——turns to social media platforms and looks at the figure of the sad girl as she emerged online as an indirect response to a popular culture overtly focused on happiness. It discusses how she appeared on primarily Tumblr and Instagram, exploring the general sad girl discourses on these platforms as well as some examples that received extra attention. These include the artist Audrey Wollen and her sad girl theory, the girl group Sad Girls Y Qué, the Instagram club Sad Girls Club, the social media brand My Therapist Says, and prominent Instagram accounts. Here I look at the critical and acritical tendencies within the figure, acknowledging both the potentially subversive aspects of the activist-oriented sad girls and the more commercialized versions of popular sad girls. This chapter explores how Tumblr sad girls might be seen as resting in sadness; how relatability is employed as a political strategy by some Instagram sad girls; the ambivalence of normalization; and the limits of using commercial social media platforms for meaningful social action. The tension between a profitable vulnerability and supportive spaces is present also here, although the supportive element is dominant in the peer-to-peer networks formed on these platforms.

The final chapter is a conclusion that discusses how, across the three sites, conversations around depression, anxiety, and general mental illness have taken shape post-2008. By tying together the constructions of mental health in magazines, among celebrities, and on social media, the conclusion highlights how a changing media landscape and neoliberal calls for self-optimization have made way for a profitable vulnerability that exists in tension with more radical understandings of psychic wellbeing.

NOTES

1. Eells, "Billie Eilish and the Triumph of the Weird;" Frost, "Meghan Markle Says She Sought Help Over Suicidal Thoughts;" Thorne, "HBO to Add Mental Health Disclaimers in Front of Select Shows;" Young, "Prince Harry says people should train 'mind and body as one' in video launching mental health tool for military."
2. Ahmed, *The Promise of Happiness*; Davies, *The happiness industry*; Gill and Orgad, "The Confidence Cult(ure);" Orgad and Gill, *Confidence Culture*.
3. Vogue.com, "Selena Gomez Gets Real About Anxiety."
4. Pugachevsky, "27 Celebrities On Dealing With Depression And Bipolar Disorder;" see Chap. 4.

5. Kliegman, "2015: The Year Mental Illness Finally Got Some Respect on TV."
6. See Chaps. 5 and 6.
7. Gill, "Postfeminist media culture;" Gill, "Post-postfeminism?;" Negra and Tasker, *Gendering the recession*; Scharff, "The Psychic Life of Neoliberalism."
8. Gill, "Postfeminist media culture;" Gill, "Culture and Subjectivity in Neoliberal and Postfeminist Times;" McRobbie, *The aftermath of feminism*; Ringrose and Walkerdine, "Regulating The Abject;" Scharff, "Gender and neoliberalism."
9. Gill, "The affective, cultural and psychic life of postfeminism;" Scharff, "The Psychic Life of Neoliberalism."
10. Banet-Weiser, *Empowered*; Dobson, *Postfeminist Digital Cultures*; Kanai, "On not taking the self seriously;" Orgad and Gill, *Confidence Culture*.
11. Dobson and Kanai, "From "can-do" girls to insecure and angry;" Orgad and Gill, "Safety valves for mediated female rage in the #MeToo era;" Wood, "Fuck the patriarchy."
12. Dobson and Kanai, "From "can-do" girls to insecure and angry," 1.
13. Orgad and Gill, "Safety valves for mediated female rage in the #MeToo era," 596.
14. Wood, "Fuck the patriarchy."
15. Traister, *Good and Mad*.
16. Cooper, *Eloquent Rage*; Lorde, *Sister outsider*.
17. Orgad and Gill, *Confidence Culture*.
18. Ibid, 4.
19. Ibid, 52.
20. McRobbie, *Feminism and the politics of resilience*.
21. Ibid, 43-44.
22. McRobbie, "Jackie Magazine," 69.
23. Duffy, *Remake, Remodel*, 3.
24. Williams, *Marxism and Literature*.
25. Projansky, *Spectacular Girls*, 21.
26. Alderton, *The aesthetics of self-harm*, 106-107.
27. A piece aptly titled "All Alone in their White Girl Pain" circulated online in August 2020, that made some poignant remarks about the acritical and exclusionary aspects of white sad girls. Among these were that the sad girl subject position was always only available for white girls to inhabit, and that the pleasure that people like Lana del Rey derive from being victimized is only truly pleasurable to those who have not actually been victimized. Hip to Waste, "All Alone in Their White Girl Pain," newsletter blog, August 1, 2020, accessed June 28, 2022, https://hiptowaste.substack.com/p/all-alone-in-their-white-girl-pain.
28. See "The People of Color and Mental Illness Photo Project," website, accessed June 23, 2022, https://www.diorvargas.com/photoproject; and Sad Girls Club, website, accessed June 23, 2022, https://sadgirlsclub.org/.

29. See Harvard, "Mental Health Muslim Communities;" Sinay, "Experiencing Racism Makes You High Risk for Mental Health Issues;" McNamara, "Legalizing Same Sex Marriage Lowered the Suicide Rates For Lesbian, Gay and Bisexual Teens."

30. Institute for Precarious Consciousness, "WE ARE ALL VERY ANXIOUS."

31. Abad-Santos, "Meghan Markle's honesty about suicidal thoughts in her Oprah interview could help others;" Frost, "Meghan Markle Says She Sought Help Over Suicidal Thoughts."

32. Orgad and Gill, *Confidence Culture*, McRobbie, *Feminism and the politics of resilience.*

33. When I started this research, Lovato had not yet come out as non-binary, and despite their current gender-queer identity, they were still a major figure in American Girl culture in the first two decades of the twenty-first century, which is why I have kept their celebrity health narrative as an example of how mental illness is configured in media culture. Blistein, "Demi Lovato Comes Out as Gender Non-Binary."

34. Projansky, *Spectacular Girls*, 21; Sedgwick, *Touching Feeling.*

35. Sedgwick, *Touching Feeling*, 125.

36. Ibid, 128.

37. Ibid, 137

38. Appignanesi, *Sad, mad and bad*; Chesler, *Women's madness*; Showalter, *The female malady.*

39. Franssen, "The celebritization of self-care;" Johnson, "Managing Mr. Monk;" Rose, *Inventing our Selves.*

40. Vigier, "The Meaning of Lana Del Rey," 2.

41. Lana del Rey, "Video Games," YouTube video, October 16, 2011, accessed June 28, 2022, https://www.youtube.com/watch?v=cE6wxDqdOV0.

42. One YouTube user even commented in March of 2020 that "This is revolutionary. Now these [sic] kind of music is common thanks to Lana. Came at a time when we had party music during school. This changed the entire music scenario." Alisa03, March, 2020, "comment on," Lana del Rey, "Video Games," Youtube video, October 16, 2011, accessed June 28, 2022, https://www.youtube.com/watch?v=cE6wxDqdOV0.

43. Schrodt, "Lana Del Rey's Feminist Problem."

44. Powers, "Lana Del Rey: Just Another Pop Star."

45. Vigier, "The Meaning of Lana Del Rey," 4.

46. Ibid, 3.

47. Watson, "How girls are finding empowerment through being sad online."

48. Alderton, *The aesthetics of self-harm*, 64.

49. Ibid, 64.

50. Ibid; Farah, "All Alone in Their White Girl Pain."

51. A 2018 study from researchers at the University of California at Irvine analyzed 500,000 popular songs released in the UK between 1985 to

2015 and classified them according to mood, showing that there was "a clear downward trend in 'happiness' and 'brightness', as well as a slight upward trend in 'sadness,'" indicating that mainstream music has become statistically sadder. Interiano et al, "Musical trends and predictability of success in contemporary songs in and out of the top charts."

52. Kanai, "Girlfriendship and sameness;" Kanai, "The best friend, the boy-friend, other girls, hot guys, and creeps;" Kanai, *Gender and Relatability in Digital Culture.*
53. Gamson, "The Unwatched Life Is Not Worth Living;" Marwick and boyd, "To see and be seen;" Marwick, "Instafame: Luxury selfies in the attention economy."
54. Coulter and Moruzi, "Woke Girls;" see Chap. 5.
55. Cvetkovich, *Depression: A Public Feeling*, 116; Cheng, *The Melancholy of Race*; Eng and Han, "Dialogue on Racial Melancholia;" Holland, *Raising the Dead*; Gilroy, *Postcolonial Melancholia*; Khanna, *Dark Continents*; Muñoz, "Feeling Brown, Feeling Down."
56. Hartman, *Lose Your Mother*, 6; see also Cvetkovich, "Depression is ordinary."
57. Rankine, "The Condition of Black Life Is One of Mourning."
58. Cvetkovich, *Depression: A Public Feeling*, 115.
59. Springer, Birch and MacLeavy, *The handbook of neoliberalism*, 2.
60. Brown, "Neo-liberalism and the End of Liberal Democracy;" Barry, Osborne, and Rose, *Foucault and political reason*; Cruikshank, "Revolutions within: self-government and self-esteem;" Lemke, "The birth of bio-politics;" Lewis, "Governmentality at work in shaping a critical geographical politics;" Rose, *Powers of Freedom.*
61. Lemke, "The birth of bio-politics," 201.
62. Foucault, *Discipline and punish*; Foucault, *The Birth of Biopolitics.*
63. Lemke, "The birth of bio-politics," 191.
64. Ibid, 201.
65. Foucault, *Ethics: Subjectivity and Truth*, 73.
66. Rose, *The politics of life itself*, 53.
67. Ibid, 54.
68. Brown, "Neo-liberalism and the End of Liberal Democracy;" Cruikshank, "Revolutions within: self-government and self-esteem;" Foucault, *The Birth of Biopolitics*; Lemke, "The birth of bio-politics;" Rose, *Inventing our Selves*; Rose, *Powers of Freedom*; Rose, *The politics of life itself.*
69. Lupton, *The Quantified Self.*
70. Du Gay, *Consumption and identity at work*, 124.
71. Brown, "Neo-liberalism and the End of Liberal Democracy," 5, italicization in original.
72. Lupton, *The Quantified Self*, 102.

73. Barbara Cruikshank's (1996) study of the self-esteem movement of the 1980s and 1990s provides a poignant and quite literal example of how the individual becomes accountable for the welfare of an entire society. In 1983 the state of California established the "Task Force to Promote Self-Esteem and Social and Personal Responsibility," marketed not only as an attempt at making people feel better about themselves, but also as a solution to social problems like poverty, crime, and gender inequality. Claiming to be a "social revolution," the movement took aim not at capitalism, patriarchy, or white supremacy, but at "the order of the self and the way we govern our selves." In this way, problems like unemployment, discrimination, and systemic violence are not to be solved by changes to social-structural factors, but by reforming citizens on an individual-subjective level. In a neoliberal society, then, the individual's self is not just her own, but part of, and in direct causality/correlation with the social body/good. Cruikshank articulates it succinctly when she says: "The line between subjectivity and subjection is crossed when I subject my self, when I align my personal goals with those set out by reformers … according to some notion of the social good." Cruikshank, "Revolutions within," 213, 235.
74. Greene and Breshears, "Biopolitical Media," 191.
75. Rose and Miller, "Political power beyond the State," 175.
76. Ibid, 175.
77. Gill, "Postfeminist media culture," 147.
78. Butler, *The Psychic Life of Power*;
79. Scharff, "The Psychic Life of Neoliberalism," 111.
80. Gill and Elias, "Beauty surveillance," 16; Gill, "Postfeminist media culture;" Gill, "Culture and Subjectivity in Neoliberal and Postfeminist Times;" Gill, "The affective, cultural and psychic life of postfeminism."
81. Banet-Weiser, *Empowered*, 13.
82. Orgad and Gill, *Confidence Culture*, 7-8.
83. Pedwell and Whitehead, "Affecting feminism," 119.
84. Gregg and Seigworth, *The Affect Theory Reader*, 9.
85. Ahmed, *The Cultural Politics of Emotion*; Ahmed, *The Promise of Happiness*; Berlant, *The Queen of America Goes to Washington City*; Berlant, *The Female Complaint*; Cvetkovich, *An archive of feeling*; Ngai, *Ugly Feelings*; Sedgwick, *Touching Feeling*.
86. Cvetkovich, *Mixed Feelings*.
87. Pedwell and Whitehead, "Affecting feminism," 121.
88. Williams, *Marxism and Literature*.
89. Ahmed, *The Promise of Happiness*, 216; see also Ahmed, *The Cultural Politics of Emotion*.
90. Hochschild, *The Managed Heart*; Gill and Kanai, "Mediating Neoliberal Capitalism."
91. Illouz, *Cold Intimacies*.

REFERENCES

Abad-Santos, Alex. "Meghan Markle's Honesty about Suicidal Thoughts in Her Oprah Interview Could Help Others." *Vox*, March 8, 2021. https://www.vox.com/22320404/meghan-markle-suicide-oprah-cbs-interview.

Ahmed, Sara. *The Cultural Politics of Emotion*. New York: Routledge, 2004.

Ahmed, Sara. *The Promise of Happiness*. Durham and London: Duke University Press, 2010.

Alderton, Zoe. *The Aesthetics of Self-Harm: The Visual Rhetoric of Online Self-Harm Communities*. London and New York: Routledge, 2018. https://doi.org/10.4324/9781315637853-2.

Banet-Weiser, Sarah. *Empowered: Popular Feminism and Popular Misogyny*. Durham and London: Duke University Press, 2018.

Barry, Andrew, Thomas Osborne, and Nikolas Rose, eds. *Foucault and Political Reason: Liberalism, Neo-Liberalism and Rationalities of Government*. Chicago and London: University of Chicago Press, 1996. https://doi.org/10.1057/9781137291622.

Berlant, Lauren. *The Queen of America Goes to Washington City: Essays on Sex and Citizenship*. Durham and London: Duke University Press, 1997.

Berlant, Lauren. *The Female Complaint: The Unfinished Business of Sentimentality in American Culture*. Durham and London: Duke University Press, 2008.

Blistein, Jon. "Demi Lovato Comes Out as Gender Non-Binary." *Rolling Stone*, May 19, 2021. https://www.rollingstone.com/music/music-news/demi-lovato-non-binary-coming-out-pronouns-1171379/.

Butler, Judith. *The Psychic Life of Power: Theories in Subjection*. Stanford, CA: Stanford University Press, 1997.

Cheng, Anne Anlin. *The Melancholy of Race: Psychoanalysis, Assimilation, and Hidden Grief*. New York: Oxford University Press, 2000.

Cooper, Brittney. *Eloquent Rage: A Black Feminist Discovers Her Superpower*. New York: St Martin's, 2018.

Coulter, Natalie, and Kristine Moruzi. "Woke Girls: From The Girl's Realm to Teen Vogue." *Feminist Media Studies* 00, no. 00 (2020): 1–15. https://doi.org/10.1080/14680777.2020.1736119.

Cruikshank, Barbara. "Revolutions within: Self-Government and Self-Esteem." In *Foucault and Political Reason: Liberalism, Neo-Liberalism and Rationalities of Government*, edited by Andrew Barry, Thomas Osborne, and Nikolas Rose, 231–51. Chicago and London: University of Chicago Press, 1996.

Cvetkovich, Ann. *Mixed Feelings: Feminism, Mass Culture, and Victorian Sensationalism*. New Brunswick, NJ: Rutgers University Press, 1992.

Cvetkovich, Ann. *An Archive of Feeling: Trauma, Sexuality and Lesbian Public Culture*. Durham and London: Duke University Press, 2003. https://doi.org/10.1177/136346070500800112.

Cvetkovich, Ann. "Depression Is Ordinary: Public Feelings and Saidiya Hartman's Lose Your Mother." *Feminist Theory* 13, no. 2 (2012a): 131–46. https://doi.org/10.1177/1464700112442641.

Cvetkovich, Ann. *Depression: A Public Feeling.* Durham and London: Duke University Press, 2012b.

Davies, William. *The Happiness Industry: How the Government and Big Business Sold Us Well-Being.* London: Verso, 2015.

Dobson, Amy Shields. *Postfeminist Digital Cultures: Femininity, Social Media, and Self-Representation.* New York: Palgrave Macmillan, 2015.

Dobson, Amy Shields, and Akane Kanai. "From 'Can-Do' Girls to Insecure and Angry: Affective Dissonances in Young Women's Post-Recessional Media." *Feminist Media Studies*, 2018, 1–16. https://doi.org/10.1080/14680777.2018.1546206.

Gay, Paul Du. *Consumption and Identity at Work.* London, Thousand Oaks, New Dehli: SAGE Publications, 1996.

Duffy, Brooke Erin. *Remake, Remodel: Women's Magazines in the Digital Age.* Urbana, Chicago and Springfield: University of Illinois Press, 2013.

Eells, Josh. "Billie Eilish and the Triumph of the Weird: Rolling Stone Cover Story." *Rolling Stone*, July 31, 2019. https://www.rollingstone.com/music/music-features/billie-eilish-cover-story-triumph-weird-863603/.

Elias, Ana Sofia, and Rosalind Gill. "Beauty Surveillance: The Digital Self-Monitoring Cultures of Neoliberalism." *European Journal of Cultural Studies* 21, no. 1 (2018): 59–77. https://doi.org/10.1177/1367549417705604.

Eng, David L & Shinhee Han. "A Dialogue on Racial Melancholia." *Psychoanalytic Dialogues* 10, no. 4 (2008): 667–700. https://doi.org/10.1080/10481881009348576.

Foucault, Michel. *Discipline and Punish.* New York: Random House LLC, 1977.

Foucault, Michel. *Ethics: Subjectivity and Truth (Essential Works of Foucault, 1954-1984, Vol. 1).* New York: The New Press, 1997.

Foucault, Michel. *The Birth of Biopolitics: Lectures at the Collège de France, 1978-1979.* New York: Picador, 2008.

Frost, Natasha. "Meghan Markle Says She Sought Help Over Suicidal Thoughts." *The New York Times*, March 7, 2021. https://www.nytimes.com/2021/03/07/world/meghan-markle-suicidal-thoughts.html.

Gamson, Joshua. "The Unwatched Life Is Not Worth Living: The Elevation of the Ordinary in Celebrity Culture." *PMLA* 126, no. 4 (2011): 1061–69.

Gill, Rosalind. "Postfeminist Media Culture: Elements of a Sensibility." *European Journal of Cultural Studies* 10, no. 2 (May 1, 2007): 147–66. https://doi.org/10.1177/1367549407075898.

Gill, Rosalind. "Culture and Subjectivity in Neoliberal and Postfeminist Times." *Subjectivity* 25 (2008): 432–45. https://doi.org/10.1057/sub.2008.28.

Gill, Rosalind. "Post-Postfeminism?: New Feminist Visibilities in Postfeminist Times." *Feminist Media Studies* 16, no. 4 (2016): 610–30. https://doi.org/10.1080/14680777.2016.1193293.

Gill, Rosalind. "The Affective, Cultural and Psychic Life of Postfeminism: A Postfeminist Sensibility 10 Years On." *European Journal of Cultural Studies* 20, no. 6 (2017): 606–26. https://doi.org/10.1177/1367549417733003.

Gill, Rosalind, and Akane Kanai. "Mediating Neoliberal Capitalism: Affect, Subjectivity and Inequality." *Journal of Communication* 68, no. 2 (2018): 318–26. https://doi.org/10.1093/joc/jqy002.

Gill, Rosalind, and Shani Orgad. "The Confidence Cult(Ure)." *Australian Feminist Studies* 30, no. 86 (2015): 324–44.

Gilroy, Paul. *Postcolonial Melancholia.* New York: Columbia University Press, 2005.

Greene, Ronald Walter, and David Breshears. "Biopolitical Media: Population, Communications International, and the Governing of Reproductive Health." In *Governing the Female Body: Gender, Health, and Networks of Power,* 186–205. Albany, NY: State University of New York Press, 2010.

Gregg, Melissa, and Gregory Seigworth. *The Affect Theory Reader.* Durham and London: Duke University Press, 2013. https://doi.org/10.1017/CBO9781107415324.004.

Hartman, Saidiya. *Lose Your Mother: A Journey Along the Atlantic Slave Route.* New York: Farrar, Straus and Giroux, 2008.

Harvard, Sarah. "Mental Health Muslim Communities." *Teen Vogue,* November 18, 2015. https://www.teenvogue.com/story/mental-health-muslim-communities.

Hochschild, Arlie Russell. *The Managed Heart: Commercialization of Human Feeling.* Berkeley, Los Angeles, London: University of California Press, 1983.

Holland, Sharon Patricia. *Raising the Dead: Readings of Death and (Black) Subjectivity.* Durham and London: Duke University Press, 2000.

Illouz, Eva. *Cold Intimacies: The Making of Emotional Capitalism.* Cambridge, UK and Malden, MA: Polity Press, 2007.

Institute for Precarious Consciousness. "WE ARE ALL VERY ANXIOUS: Six Theses on Anxiety and Why It Is Effectively Preventing Militancy, and One Possible Strategy for Overcoming It." *Weareplanc.Org,* April 4, 2014. https://www.weareplanc.org/blog/we-are-all-very-anxious/.

Interiano, Myra, Kamyar Kazemi, Lijia Wang, Jienian Yang, Zhaoxia Yu, and Natalia L. Komarova. "Musical Trends and Predictability of Success in Contemporary Songs in and out of the Top Charts." *Royal Society Open Science* 5, no. 5 (2018). https://doi.org/10.1098/rsos.171274.

Kanai, Akane. "The Best Friend, the Boyfriend, Other Girls, Hot Guys, and Creeps: The Relational Production of Self on Tumblr." *Feminist Media Studies* 17, no. 6 (2017a): 911–25. https://doi.org/10.1080/14680777.2017.1298647.

Kanai, Akane. "Girlfriendship and Sameness: Affective Belonging in a Digital Intimate Public." *Journal of Gender Studies* 26, no. 3 (2017b): 293–306. https://doi.org/10.1080/09589236.2017.1281108.

Kanai, Akane. *Gender and Relatability in Digital Culture: Managing Affect, Intimacy and Value*. Cham: Palgrave Macmillan, 2019a. https://doi.org/10.1007/978-3-319-91515-9.

Kanai, Akane. "On Not Taking the Self Seriously: Resilience, Relatability and Humour in Young Women's Tumblr Blogs." *European Journal of Cultural Studies* 22, no. 1 (2019b): 60–77. https://doi.org/10.1177/1367549417722092.

Khanna, Ranjana. *Dark Continents: Psychoanalysis and Colonialism*. Durham: Duke University Press, 2003.

Kliegman, Julie. "2015: The Year Mental Illness Finally Got Some Respect on TV." *Vulture.Com*, December 18, 2015. http://www.vulture.com/2015/12/mental-illness-got-some-respect-on-tv-in-2015.html.

Lemke, Thomas. "'The Birth of Bio-Politics': Michel Foucault's Lecture at the Collège de France on Neo-Liberal Governmentality." *Economy and Society* 30, no. 2 (2001): 190–207. https://doi.org/10.1080/03085140120042271.

Lewis, Nick. "Governmentality at Work in Shaping a Critical Geographical Politics." In *The Handbook of Neoliberalism*, edited by Simon Springer, Kean Birch, and Julie MacLeavy, 73–83. Oxon, UK and New York, USA: Routledge, 2016.

Lorde, Audre. *Sister Outsider: Essays and Speeches*. New York: The Crossing Press Feminist Series, 1984.

Lupton, Deborah. *The Quantified Self: A Sociology of Self-Tracking*. Cambridge, UK and Malden, MA: Polity Press, 2016.

McNamara, Brittney. "Legalizing Same Sex Marriage Lowered the Suicide Rates For Lesbian, Gay and Bisexual Teens." *Teen Vogue*, February 21, 2017. https://www.teenvogue.com/story/same-sex-marriage-lowered-suicide-rate.

McRobbie, Angela. "Jackie Magazine: Romantic Individualism and the Teenage Girl." In *Feminism and Youth Culture*, 2nd ed. New York: Routledge, 2000.

McRobbie, Angela. *The Aftermath of Feminism: Gender, Culture and Social Change*. London, Thousand Oaks, New Delhi and Singapore: SAGE, 2009.

McRobbie, Angela. *Feminism and the Politics of Resilience: Essays on Gender, Media and the End of Welfare*. Cambridge and Medford: Polity Press, 2020.

Muñoz, José Esteban. "Feeling Brown, Feeling down: Latina Affect, the Performativity of Race, and the Depressive Position." *Signs* 31, no. 3 (March 19, 2006): 675–88. https://doi.org/10.1086/499080/ASSET/IMAGES/LARGE/FG1_ONLINE.JPEG.

Negra, Diane, and Yvonne Tasker, eds. *Gendering the Recession: Media and Culture in an Age of Austerity*. Durham and London: Duke University Press, 2014.

Ngai, Sianne. *Ugly Feelings*. Cambridge, MA and London, England: Harvard University Press, 2005.

Orgad, Shani, and Rosalind Gill. "Safety Valves for Mediated Female Rage in the #MeToo Era." *Feminist Media Studies* 19, no. 4 (2019): 596–603. https://doi.org/10.1080/14680777.2019.1609198.

Orgad, Shani, and Rosalind Gill. *Confidence Culture.* Durham and London: Duke University Press, 2022. https://doi.org/10.1215/9781478021834.

Pedwell, Carolyn, and Anne Whitehead. "Affecting Feminism: Questions of Feeling in Feminist Theory." *Feminist Theory* 13, no. 2 (2012): 115–29. https://doi.org/10.1177/1464700112442635.

Powers, Ann. "Lana Del Rey: Just Another Pop Star." *Npr.Org*, January 30, 2012. https://www.npr.org/sections/therecord/2012/01/31/146088800/putting-together-the-pieces-of-lana-del-rey.

Projansky, Sarah. *Spectacular Girls: Media Fascination and Celebrity Culture.* New York & London: New York University Press, 2014.

Pugachevsky, Julia. "27 Celebrities On Dealing With Depression And Bipolar Disorder." *BuzzFeed*, November 7, 2014. https://www.buzzfeed.com/julia-pugachevsky/celebrities-on-dealing-with-depression-and-bipolar-disord.

Rankine, Claudia. "The Condition of Black Life Is One of Mourning." *New York Times*, June 22, 2015. https://www.nytimes.com/2015/06/22/magazine/the-condition-of-black-life-is-one-of-mourning.html.

Ringrose, Jessica, and Valerie Walkerdine. "Regulating The Abject: The TV Makeover as Site of Neo-Liberal Reinvention toward Bourgeois Femininity." *Feminist Media Studies* 8, no. 3 (2008): 227–46. https://doi.org/10.1080/14680770802217279.

Rose, Nikolas. *Inventing Our Selves: Psychology, Power, and Personhood.* Cambridge, New York and Melbourne: Cambridge University Press, 1998.

Rose, Nikolas. *Powers of Freedom: Framing Political Thought.* Cambridge, UK: Cambridge University Press, 2004. https://doi.org/10.1017/CBO9781107415324.004.

Rose, Nikolas. *The Politics of Life Itself.* Princeton University Press, 2007.

Scharff, Christina. "Gender and Neoliberalism: Young Women as Ideal Neoliberal Subjects." In *The Handbook of Neoliberalism*, edited by Simon Spring, Kean Birch, and Julie MacLeavy, 217–26. London: Routledge, 2016a.

Scharff, Christina. "The Psychic Life of Neoliberalism: Mapping the Contours of Entrepreneurial Subjectivity." *Theory, Culture & Society* 33, no. 6 (2016b): 107–22. https://doi.org/10.1177/0263276415590164.

Schrodt, Paul. "Lana Del Rey's Feminist Problem." *Slant Magazine*, February 8, 2012. https://www.slantmagazine.com/music/lana-del-reys-feminist-problem/.

Sedgwick, Eve Kosofsky. *Touching Feeling: Affect, Pedagogy, Performativity.* Durham and London: Duke University Press, 2003.

Sinay, Danielle. "Experiencing Racism Makes You High Risk for Mental Health Issues." *Teen Vogue*, August 2, 2016. https://www.teenvogue.com/story/racism-mental-health-distress-study.

Springer, Simon, Kean Birch, and Julie Macleavy. *The Handbook of Neoliberalism.* Oxon, UK and New York, USA: Routledge, 2016.

Thorne, Will. "HBO to Add Mental Health Disclaimers in Front of Select Shows." *Variety*, October 10, 2019. https://variety.com/2019/tv/news/hbo-mental-health-awareness-banner-1203365233/.

Traister, Rebecca. *Good and Mad: The Revolutionary Power of Women's Anger.* New York: Simon & Schuster, 2018.

Vargas, Dior. "POC & Mental Illness Photo Project." Accessed May 15, 2020. http://diorvargas.com/poc-mental-illness/.

Vigier, Catherine. "The Meaning of Lana Del Rey: Pop Culture, Post-Feminism and the Choices Facing Young Women Today." *Zeteo: The Journal of Interdisciplinary Writing*, no. Fall (2012): 1–16.

Vogue.com. "Selena Gomez Gets Real About Anxiety—And How Therapy Changed Everything." *Vogue.Com*, March 16, 2017. https://www.vogue.com/article/selena-gomez-rehab-therapy-mental-health-depression.

Williams, Raymond. *Marxism and Literature.* Oxford: Oxford University Press, 1977.

Wood, Helen. "Fuck the Patriarchy: Towards an Intersectional Politics of Irreverent Rage." *Feminist Media Studies* 19, no. 4 (2019): 609–15. https://doi.org/10.1080/14680777.2019.1609232.

Young, Sarah. "Prince Harry Says People Should Train 'mind and Body as One' in Video Launching Mental Health Tool for Military." *The Independent*, April 27, 2020. https://www.independent.co.uk/life-style/royal-family/prince-harry-headfit-military-soldier-mental-health-tool-video-heads-together-a9485771.html.

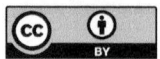

CHAPTER 2

A Historical Lineage of Sad and Mad Women

Women's affective states have a long history of being pathologized under names like neurasthenia, hysteria, and schizophrenia.[1] In culture, the sad and mad woman has appeared as various popular figures: the Victorian madwoman, the hysteric, the schizophrenic, and the Prozac-consuming American woman of the 1990s, to name a few. The question of how specific pathologizations relate to contemporary gender relations runs through all of these iterations of mad and sad women. Some feminist scholars have argued that definitions of mental illness have been directly linked to conventional understandings of femininity and masculinity, and that any norm violation has been understood as madness.[2] And others have pointed to the biological reactions of some historical patients to highlight the "realness" of their symptoms.[3]

In this chapter I trace a brief history of how women's mental health has been pathologized in the American and European West. I hope to show that mental illness diagnoses are neither completely discursive (socially and linguistically constructed) nor fixed neurological truths (biological facts of life that always look the same), but emerge and take shape in a complex interplay between sociocultural discourses and an ever-developing medical science.

In charting this brief history I draw heavily on scholars like Elaine Showalter and Lisa Appignanesi who mark the turn from the eighteen to the nineteenth century (1700 to 1800) as the start of the modern conception of mental illness and health in distinctively gendered ways.[4] This turn of the century is significant for multiple reasons, one of them of course

© The Author(s) 2023
F. Thelandersson, *21st Century Media and Female Mental Health*,
https://doi.org/10.1007/978-3-031-16756-0_2

being the dawn of Enlightenment ideas and the birth of the human sciences that introduced new ways of organizing the world and knowledge about it. The decades around the French revolution marks an epistemic shift in medicines, sciences, and penitentiary systems of the West.

Here I follow Foucault's conceptualization of the epistemological shift of this turn of the century, which when it came to penitentiary systems, involved a move from punishing the body of the criminal to disciplining the soul.[5] According to Foucault, the change in the judicial system from publicly torturing its criminals to confining them with the purpose of rehabilitating or "curing" them, only had the appearance of being more humane. The control exercised over the individual through the enactment of disciplinary practices is just as efficient, if not more so, than the control of the body, because it initiates a deeper and more long-lasting grip on the soul. When self-discipline has been properly internalized (supposedly in a successful process of rehabilitation), the powers that be have a hold on the individual, who will adjust his behavior in accordance to what best suits the dominant power structures. The concepts of governmentality and bio-politics that were developed later in Foucault's career build on these analyses of penitentiary systems. Governmentality furthers our understanding of how the internalization of discipline works and takes hold of the individual at the level of subject formation. In relation to mental health and illness, governmentality allows us to think about how the social/political affects the organization of our psyches.

Foucault also delineates this shift from "outwardly" to inwardly discipline in relation to sexuality and madness. In broad strokes, what is described here is how views and conceptualizations of the criminal, the mad, and the abnormal came to be constructed within the "new" human sciences in post-Enlightenment Europe.[6] A "medical gaze" was being established in the new medical clinics, and the mad were to be not just managed but also understood.[7] Crucial to this was the establishment of a firm binary between reason and unreason, civilized and uncivilized. The poles in this binary were presented as objectively true, free of any agendas. Part of this new knowledge regime was the establishment of sciences that "uncovered" already existing truths. What Foucault so crucially showed was that these new epistemologies were not simple discoveries of a firm and already existing order of things, but were in themselves acts of ordering things.

In regard to psychology and psychiatry this meant the establishment of a field of knowledge which could display an ultimate picture of how the psyche functions and subsequently prescribe it treatments to cure or better its makeup. But looking at the history of these disciplines, it quickly becomes clear that the truth that it has presented as absolute has contingently changed with contemporary power structures.

The Victorian Madwoman

One of the most significant changes brought on by the "new" epistemology of the psyche at the turn of the century was the move from the lunatic-as-animal to the lunatic-as-human, from nonperson to person. Where the mad had previously been seen as "unfeeling brutes, ferocious animals that needed to be kept in check with chains," they were now regarded as sick human beings who might be returned to sanity under the correct care.[8]

This shift affected both popular imagination and actual practices of caring for the mentally ill. As a result of this ideological change English social reformers began to build asylums "in which paternal surveillance and religious ideals replaced physical coercion, fear and force."[9] The attitude toward, and treatment of, the mentally ill thus went from being one of sensational disgust to protective pity. Just as the criminal justice system underwent an overhaul from public punishments like torture and executions to "sophisticated" retributions aimed at rehabilitation, so the psychiatric establishment went from shunning the mad as definite outcasts to treating them as patients in need and in hope of saving.

Importantly, Showalter positions this shift next to another ideological change, when "the dialectic of reason and unreason took on specifically sexual meanings, and … the symbolic gender of the insane person shifted from male to female."[10] Reason became synonymous with men and masculinity and unreason with women and femininity. In the move toward less violent and more reparative care of the mentally ill, the subject in need of caring confinement became primarily female, and the treatment of her was in the hands of men and male doctors. In this way, the shift in psychiatric care was one of many arenas in which rationality became associated with men and irrationality with women. It was the rationally sound mind that had the capacity to control and cure the irrationally mad one.

Showalter describes the change in the symbolic conceptualization of the lunatic in the eighteenth century: "in the course of the century … the appealing madwoman gradually displaced the repulsive madman, both as a prototype of the confined lunatic and as a cultural icon."[11] Showalter illustrates this change in cultural perception by showcasing two statues of mad*men* that had represented the figure of lunacy from the seventeenth century on, but were removed from the public by the early nineteenth century. Caius Gabriel Cibber's statues "Raving Madness" and "Melancholy Madness" (both made in 1677), depicted two men in the nude, half-lying on the ground, one aggravated and bound in shackles and the other in an infantilized position of weakness. The statues were placed at the entrance of the Bethlem (known as Bedlam) Hospital in London, one of the first and most notorious asylums in England. These statues were the most famous representations of madness at the time. Showalter describes them as marking "the lunatic's entrance into the netherworld of the insane."[12] But in 1815 the statues in front of Bedlam were replaced by figures of women, representing "a youthful, beautiful, female insanity."[13] From now on, the representation of madness "was becoming feminized and tamed, no longer wild, raving and dangerous, but pathetic."[14] The popular image of psychic ills was no longer that of a madman, but of a madwoman.

One part of this shift was the prevalence of stories of frail women being mistreated in asylums, which reached the public and changed the opinion about the treatment of the mad toward the end of the eighteenth century, inspiring legal and institutional reforms.[15] For example, Showalter recounts the story of a Quaker widow who died under inexplicable circumstances in the York asylum, resulting in the official outrage of a wealthy philanthropist who started the York retreat, "an asylum that pioneered the humane care of the insane."[16] This illustration implies that the victimized madwomen who inspired public concern belonged primarily to the upper middle class. Perhaps not unsurprisingly, the abuse of the wealthy attracted more attention than the mistreatment of the ostracized poor. But in accordance with the newfound rational value of human life, the penniless were not shut out from the compassionate treatment of the mad, they were just carefully segregated within the institutions.

Patients were geographically separated within the asylum based on gender and class. The intellectual rehabilitation activities created for the patients were also divided by class, with the richer clientele being treated to lectures by local experts on poetry and biology, while the "paupers" were left to lecture each other.[17] Class structures were thus deliberately reproduced down to a tangible and material level. The insane of all classes could be cured, but no illusions of social mobility were allowed to take hold. In accordance with what Showalter calls "psychiatric Darwinism," which appointed biological and genetic predispositions as causes of mental illness, the notion that mental health could correspond to socioeconomic status was completely ignored.

One of the most popular diagnoses during the Victorian era was also closely tied to class. Neurasthenia, coined in 1869 by George M. Beard, referred to "the morbid condition of the exhaustion of the nervous system" and grew out of the "American way of life, with its race for money and power, its excessive pursuit of capital and technological progress."[18] It was often middle-class women who dared to pursue "masculine" activities like intellectual thinking who received the diagnosis, which followed an idea of the nervous system as possessing a finite amount of nervous energy that could more easily be depleted than replenished. The demands of the new world could easily exhaust women's frail nerves and the cure prescribed was often a totalizing rest that urged the patient to abstain from all activity, exercise, and work. Charlotte Perkins Gilman's now classic novel *The Yellow Wallpaper* (1892) depicts the experience of fulfilling such a cure, and exemplifies how the very rest ordained to calm the nerves could be what furthers the patient's descent into madness.

Socially mobile middle-class women thus found themselves in a double bind, where the culture at large championed dynamism and speed, but demanded that women comply and acquiesce. As a response to these contradictions, women frequently developed "nervous troubles which the doctors then linked to their specifically female functions rather than to the overall conditions of their lives."[19]

Ophelia, Crazy Jane, and Lucia

In Victorian England the madwoman was culturally and artistically represented and perpetuated in three major forms: as "the suicidal Ophelia, the sentimental Crazy Jane, and the violent Lucia."[20] Ophelia, the love-interest of Shakespeare's Hamlet, "goes mad" and drowns herself after finding out that her potential husband has killed her father. Showalter describes the two other figures as derivations of Ophelia. Crazy Jane was the recurring fictional figure of a penniless maid who "goes mad" when her lover leaves her. She was "a touching image of feminine vulnerability and a flattering reminder of female dependence upon male affection."[21] If Crazy Jane represented an unthreatening female madness, a mostly passive yearning for love gone wrong, Lucia or Lucy was her vicious antonym that embodied "female sexuality as insane violence against men."[22] Originating from Walter Scott's novel *The Bride of Lammermoor* (1819), Lucy had had to give up on the man she loved to marry another, and on the wedding night she "goes mad" and brutally murders her new husband. Lucy's story became a wildly popular theme in nineteenth-century opera, coming to represent a female flight from the shackles of contemporary femininity. The violent madness she fled into was seen by some feminists as an empowering moment that the female opera-goer could experience indirectly, thus herself feeling a sense of liberation from her confined everyday existence.

The idea that a fictional female character gone mad could function as a moment of empowering identification for the contemporary woman appears in multiple feminist readings of women and madness in the cultural imaginary. Sandra Gilbert and Susan Gubar's *The Madwoman in the Attic* is perhaps the most famous work to argue such a stance. Referencing Mr Rochester's wife who is hidden away in the attic in *Jane Eyre*, Gilbert and Gubar interpreted her as "the author's double, an image of her own anxiety and rage" against patriarchy.[23]

Gilbert and Gubar defined a female literary tradition in nineteenth-century writing and discerned a recurring theme of psychological ailments across genres and geographical locations. Some of the recurring tropes were images of "enclosure and escape, fantasies in which maddened doubles functioned as asocial surrogates for docile selves, metaphors of physical discomfort manifested in frozen landscapes and fiery interiors … along with obsessive depictions of diseases like anorexia, agoraphobia, and claustrophobia."[24] Rather than reading this as a simple reflection of the reality of female lives at the time, Gilbert and Gubar see the narratives of madness as ways in which the authors could symbolically act out a refusal of patriarchal norms. The character on the page functioned as the author's double, enabling her to express dissatisfaction and rage at the conventions she had limited capacities to protest in everyday life.

Gilbert and Gubar's text has taken an almost canonical position in feminist literary scholarship, inspiring numerous analyses of female narratives of madness as radically empowering. In this framework female "madness signified anger and therefore, by extension, protest."[25] But it has also inspired critiques such as Marta Caminero-Santangelo's *The Madwoman Can't Speak: Or Why Insanity is Not Subversive*.

Caminero-Santangelo shows that the glorified figure of the madwoman, whether she's fragile and in need of saving or self-destructively and outwardly violent, is almost always white. The privilege of adopting a "mad" persona to protest a patriarchal structure is primarily awarded to white, middle-class women. In response to countless feminist readings of white women's stories, she brings in works by women of color writers like Toni Morrison, Helena Maria Viramontes, and Cristina García to diversify the analysis of "madness-narratives."[26]

Drawing on Toni Morrison's *The Bluest Eye, Sula,* and *Beloved,* Caminero-Santangelo argues that madness, rather than being subversive, may actually be seen as a capitulation to an oppressive hegemony. The act of "going mad" might function as a rebellious "giving up" on the expectations placed upon you by a male-dominated world for the white Bourgeois subject. But for the nonwhite subject, "going mad" is not a refusal of outside expectations, it is a fulfillment of them. For the protagonists in Morrison's novels, "madness consists not of subversion but rather of surrender to the representations of others; madness constitutes the inability to construct a counternarrative of any sort."[27] This racial bias can be seen in the contemporary representations of mental illness as well, where the subject who speaks openly about her troubles tends to be white and middle or upper class, and posits some level of respectability.

THE FRENCH HYSTERIC AT THE SALPÊTRIÈRE

In Paris in the early nineteenth century, the physician Philippe Pinel opened the Salpêtrière hospital "as an asylum in the modern sense, whose first principle was the *treatment* of madness."[28] The mad were not only to be confined or handled, but also to be understood and taken care of, which was a novel approach at the time.

Pinel himself has been given almost cult-like status in the history of (French) psychiatry due to his role after the Revolution in unchaining "the lunatics at the Bicêtre and the Salpêtrière, a politically symbolic act like the freeing of the prisoners in the Bastille."[29] He is shown in Tony Robert-Fleury's painting "Pinel Freeing the Insane" (1876) which depicts multiple madwomen being unshackled under the oversight of Pinel. This painting represents "the turning point ... which Pinel is said to have effected in the mythology of madness."[30] The painting hung in the lecture hall of the Salpêtrière where Jean-Martin Charcot conducted his now infamous public lectures on hysteria. During the winter of 1885–1886 Sigmund Freud attended these lectures and in writing about them mentioned the painting, describing it as a reminder of the revolutionary aspects of treating the mentally ill.[31] The anecdote of this one art piece illustrates not only the influence of Pinel, but also the far-reaching ambitions of the new humane psychiatry or "moral therapy." Like the change in the penal system from physical punishment to mental discipline, the mad were to be freed from the status of prisoners and become patients possible to cure.

Showalter's reading of "Pinel Freeing the Insane" calls out the gendered nature of the operation—men representing the voice of reason, able to free and help the irrational and helpless madwomen. This is the same mechanism as in the shift in England from the lunatic being exemplified by a repulsive man to a victimized woman. The new lunatic was a hysteric woman who could be cured by a male doctor. Under the guise of a more humane and rational approach to the mad, a new epistemology of madness was established.

At the Salpêtrière the methods by which this new body of knowledge was "uncovered" was particularly interesting because its main protagonist—neurologist Jean-Martin Charcot—made use of visual materials and photography to establish the bulk of his scholarship. The role of visual performance at the Salpêtrière was exemplified in Charcot's weekly public lectures in which he hypnotized patients in front of an audience to illustrate the different phases of hysteria, and in the rigorous photographic documentation of his work. He even had a photographer set up residency in the hospital, complete with a studio to capture the attacks of the hysterics.[32] In this way the notion of hysteria was from the beginning an extremely mediated one, it existed in its purest form only in front of an audience or a camera.

Hysteria: A Female Ailment

Hysteria is one of the psychological ailments most connected to the female gender in the Western cultural imaginary. The Salpêtrière had a special wing for male hysterics, but this fact has not survived in the popular imagination, and its male manifestation was largely reconceptualized as shell shock after World War I.[33] The word hysteria is even derived from the Greek and Latin word for uterus or womb, reflecting the long-held notion that it was caused by the female reproductive organs.[34] Georges Didi-Huberman suggests that hysteria (in the nineteenth century) was the symptom *"of being a woman."*[35] He recounts how Freud, in 1888, described hysteria as a "bête noire"—a thing that one highly dislikes, is even disgusted by; it "represented a *great fear* for everyone."[36] These were the sentiments that fueled the male doctors' studies of hysteria, and they reveal a simultaneous fear, disgust, and fascination with not only the disease, but also the entire female reproduction system. Didi-Huberman explains: "The *bête noire* was a secret and at the same time an excess. The *bête noire* was a dirty trick of feminine desire, its most shameful part ... Hysteria almost never stopped calling the feminine *guilty*."[37] Didi-Huberman thus connects hysteria to the very definition of femininity, suggesting that the diagnosis itself was part of male fear of female sexuality.

Charcot's major contribution was a psychological theory of hysteria, which held that the disease was caused by emotion, but manifested itself in actual physical symptoms. He 'proved', "through careful observation, physical examination, and the use of hypnosis ... that hysterical symptoms ... were genuine, and not under the conscious control of the patient."[38]

Didi-Huberman delineates how Charcot took the multiple expressions of hysteria, such as "spasms, convulsions, blackouts, semblances of epilepsy, catalepsies, ecstasies, comas, lethargies, deliria," assigned them an order and combined them into "a general type that can be called 'the great hysterical attack'."[39] He defined four stages of this attack: "the epileptoid phase," which resembled an epileptic seizure; "clownism," which involved exaggerated contortions; "attitudes passionnelles," in which the patient reenacted events and emotions from her life; and "delirium," when the patient starts hallucinating and talk incoherently.[40]

The stages of the complete attack were displayed in Charcot's public lectures, in which he brought in a patient, hypnotized her, and simulated the various phases for the audience to see. These lectures were attended by a diverse collection of people, not only medical students but authors, journalists, actors, and socialites. One of the recurring patients was Blanche Wittman, who was particularly good at displaying the various phases of the attack. She gained celebrity status as one of Charcot's "star hysterics."[41] There was a performative element in these displays, but to what degree the patients consciously emulated the movements that were expected of them is unclear. Showalter points out that the patients were surrounded by images of how hysterical attacks were supposed to play out, which influenced their performance under hypnosis.

The Role of Photography

At the time of Charcot's glory days at the Salpêtrière photography was making its entrance on the world scene as the true depicter of "objective reality." Didi-Huberman writes that photography "always says more than the best description; and, where medicine is concerned, it seemed to fulfill *the very ideal of the 'Observation'.*"[42] This trust in the medium made photography "the paradigm of the scientist's 'true retina'" during the nineteenth century.[43] To photographically record the research on hysteria that Charcot was undertaking was thus an obvious decision. Through photography the essence of hysteria was to be documented and categorized, to be made part of a proper science.

One of the (many) things about this that seem remarkable today is the way this documentation took place. For example, the photographic technology of the time was not sophisticated enough to snap an image immediately, meaning that the patients had to hold the pose that displayed their hysteric symptoms for the entirety of the exposure time, which could be several minutes long.[44]

The photographs of Charcot's patients were compiled into three volumes of a book titled *Photographic Iconography of the Salpêtrière (Iconographie photographique de la Salpêtrière)* (1875-1880).[45] The star patient of the Iconography was Augustine, a 15-year-old girl who had had her first hysterical attack at age 13, after being raped by her employer who was also her mother's lover.[46]

Augustine appears in multiple photographs in the Iconography, displaying all the stages of the hysterical attack, as well as variations on the expressions of each phase (see Fig. 2.1). Showalter describes Augustine as the perfect hysteric for Charcot's methods. Emphasizing the performative aspects of the photographic documentation, she states that "among her gifts was her ability to time and divide her hysterical performances into scenes, acts, tableaux, and intermissions, to perform on cue and on schedule with the click of the camera."[47]

If the madwoman in England during the nineteenth century was embodied by Ophelia and Crazy Jane, in France she was represented by Charcot's hysterics at the Salpêtrière, among them Augustine. In one sense Ophelia and Augustine were fundamentally different—the former being fictional and the latter an actual young woman sent to Charcot for treatment. But the sensational nature of Augustine's case made her more of a cultural figure than an individual person. She was and is the prime example of nineteenth-century hysteria, an icon of this stage in the "mythology of madness." This is probably why her case has been studied so frequently by feminist scholars, many reading it as a male doctor manipulating a young woman to perform symptoms to support his theories,[48] and others as a complex mix of "real" and made-up symptoms.[49]

Fig. 2.1 Augustine displaying one stage of the hysteric attack, *Iconographie photographique de la Salpêtrière.*

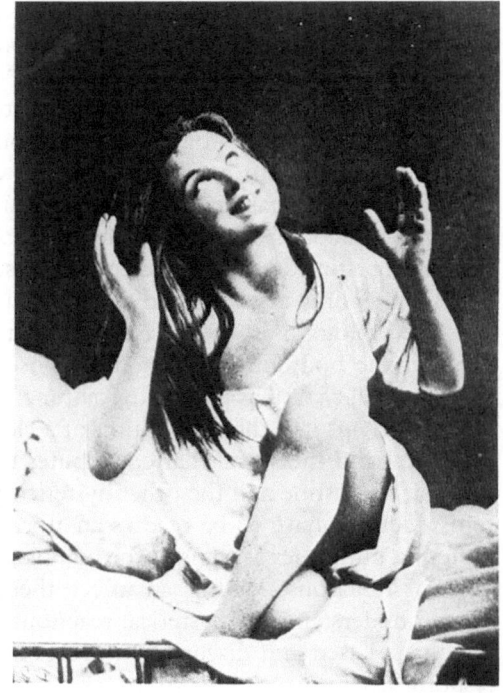

Planche XXIII

ATTITUDES PASSIONNELLES

EXTASE (1878).

Feminism and Hysteria

Showalter's stance on the male influence on hysterics has been critiqued as overtly simplistic by scholars like Elizabeth A. Wilson, who calls out Showalter for ignoring the biological aspects of "madwomen." Wilson calls Showalter's analysis of hysteria an example of "the manner in which a retreat from biology became naturalized early in the feminist interest in hysteria."[50] Describing Showalter's analysis of Charcot's treatment of hysteria as a simple suppression of female resistance, Wilson points out that some of the physical ailments suffered by the hysterics are too complex to be dismissed as socially constructed symptoms. Wilson focuses on an event in which Augustine temporarily lost the ability to see color, instead seeing everything in black and white. Showalter's analysis argues that this occurrence was a result of Charcot's sensationalist photographic methods, which finally "took its toll on her psyche."[51] Wilson counters this conclusion by asking "what kind of biological material ... stops processing color under the sway of a photographic seduction? Why is the astonishment of Augustine's symptom attributed only to Charcot and not also to the remarkable, hysterical vicissitudes of Augustine's eyes and brain?"[52]

A photograph from the *Photographic Iconography of the Salpêtrière* shows Augustine's body, stiff as a board, suspended between two chairs that support only her head and feet.[53] Such imagery makes it hard to dismiss the biological aspects of hysteria. Instances like this, where hysteria contorts the body into unimaginable poses, warrant examination of the physiological as well as psychological functions involved.

But perhaps it is the assumption of a clear differentiation between the biological and the social that contributes to both of these readings. The fact that Augustine and the other hysterics developed physiological symptoms does not have to be read as an affirmation of the "reality" of their hysterias, but rather as signs of the complex interplay between mental and physical functions. Within an affect theoretical framework, we might instead understand the hysterical reactions as examples of how the social (language-based and discursive) impacts us at the level of our biological responses.

THE BIRTH OF PSYCHOANALYSIS

The hysterics at the Salpêtrière often shared a sexually traumatized past and lived a highly sexually charged present. Charcot did not focus explicitly on this aspect of the disorder, but his most famous student, Freud, tried to understand the sexual genesis of the condition and placed conflicted sexuality at the root of severe illness.[54] Inspired by Charcot, Freud's early case histories share many similarities with the hysterics of the Salpêtrière. But whereas Charcot did not listen to what the female patients had to say and favored experimental treatment with hypnosis, pressure techniques, and drugs, Freud paid attention to how they themselves talked about their afflictions.[55] Freud and his mentor Josef Breuer pioneered the psychoanalytic treatment of hysteria with the case of Anna O. With her, dialogue took the place of observation. Instead of detached examination Breuer and Freud talked directly to the hysteric. They concluded that Anna O's hysterical symptoms were reactions to her oppressive, traditional, upbringing and lack of intellectual stimulation. The cure that Breuer prescribed was daily talking and listening, an early form of psychoanalysis.[56]

Breuer and Freud thus placed the cause of hysteria more in social circumstances than in biological predisposition. Showalter writes that they appeared "to lay the groundwork for a culturally aware therapy that took women's words and women's lives seriously, that respected the aspirations of New Women, and that allowed women a say in the management of hysterical symptoms."[57] It seemed that the introduction of talk-based therapy allowed women who suffered hysteric symptoms to finally speak for themselves and articulate their own thoughts and emotions.

With Charcot the unconscious began to be theorized, and with Freud and his contemporaries at the turn of the twentieth century it took on "a key role in understanding both madness and ordinary everyday behaviour," restructuring the way we understand the human psyche and subjectivity.[58] With the advent of psychoanalysis, a language of psychosexuality was established at a time when sexuality became increasingly important in Western lives. One's sexuality was a key indicator of the kind of person one was, normal or perverted, sane or mad. And as Foucault has shown, this organizing principle of subjectivity often involved a problematization of the sexuality of women, homosexuals, and children.[59] Ideas about sexual repression, the unconscious and the family were circulating among several scholars in the early days of the twentieth century, but "what Freud gradually and magnificently added was a narrative and theories which provided pattern, motive forces and surprising explanations that did away with moralizing punishments and liberated sexuality."[60] For Freud, contemporary sexual morality, lack of libidinal satisfaction and ignorance about sex, produced anxiety and illness. The problem, in other words, was the repressing mores of society rather than inherent vices. Freud also crucially showed that conflicts of sexuality in childhood not only shaped those who suffered enough to find their way to the couch of a psychoanalyst, but also affected all individuals, even the presumably "healthy" ones.[61]

The cultural image of the madwoman changed as well. The upper middle-class or wealthy woman who was sent to (or voluntarily visited) the psychoanalytic clinic was very different from the working-class woman interned at the Salpêtrière. Anna O. came from a wealthy, Orthodox Jewish, family. Her brother was sent off to university while the intellectually gifted Anna had to stay home and tend to domestic chores. Several of Freud's patients at the time had similar backgrounds and intellectual abilities. His and Breuer's theory was that it was the culture which confined these women to the boredom of domestic life that caused their hysteria. Within this framework the hysteric was not a fascinatingly repulsive and incontrollable figure, like at the Salpêtrière, but a likeable and admired one.[62] Compare the social circumstances of Freud and Breuer's hysterics to Augustine's. The latter was a live-in maid in a wealthy household, whose head patriarch sexually abused her at age 13.[63] Both of these social circumstances support a theory of social and cultural context as causes of hysteria, but it is telling that the view of the hysteric as sympathetic and admirable is only awarded to the wealthy one.

From Hysteric to Schizophrenic

The fascination with hysteria largely faded in the period after World War II, with schizophrenia taking its place. Statistically, schizophrenia did not primarily afflict women, as hysteria did, but was equally prevalent in women and men. This did not affect the fact that the figure of the female schizophrenic in mid-twentieth-century culture became what the hysteric was in nineteenth-century culture. Showalter explains that "modernist literary movements have appropriated the schizophrenic woman as the symbol of linguistic, religious, and sexual breakdown and rebellion." This is why, for Showalter, the disease "offers a remarkable example of the cultural conflation of femininity and insanity."[64]

Some schizophrenic symptoms, particularly "passivity, depersonalization, disembodiment, and fragmentation" have been read as a direct reflection of women's social situation. Some feminist scholars have argued that schizophrenia is the perfect literary metaphor for the female condition, expressive of women's lack of confidence, dependency on external, often masculine, definitions of the self, split between the body as sexual object and the mind as subject, and vulnerability to conflicting social messages about femininity and maturity.[65]

Within this framework it is society's patriarchal structures that are to blame when a woman becomes schizophrenic. Similar to the early Freudian analyses of hysteria, it is the limited roles available to women that cause the disease. In many of the literary works from the early 1960s that deal with schizophrenia, the act of institutionalizing women on the grounds of their diagnosis is represented as patriarchy's way of attempting to control women who do not conform.[66]

One of the most known and lauded literary heroines associated with schizophrenia is Sylvia Plath. Her fictional work *The Bell Jar* (1963) inspired many feminist readings of the protagonist as breaking down under the pressures of patriarchal society. With Plath's real life following a very similar trajectory, and ending in suicide at age 30, she was established as an icon of contemporary female madness. Part of a larger movement of female literature critical of contemporary psychiatric institutions, she also became an important figure in the early women's liberation movement of the 1960s. For the American feminist movement at the time, Plath "grew into a saint of female victimization, her madness and suicide themselves signals of what patriarchy did to talented women who dared to aspire."[67]

During the 1950s and 60s, schizophrenia became the most common diagnosis in America, and shortened in everyday speech to "schizzy" it became a synonym for crazy, odd, weird, or peculiar.[68] Many of the behaviors that were diagnosed as pathological at the time would most likely be understood as defiance or teenage unruliness today, and this over-diagnostication fueled feminist interpretations of schizophrenia as something used to limit women with aspirations beyond contemporary gender conventions.[69]

Feminism and Psychoanalysis

While Freud himself most likely had no moralizing intentions behind his work, when psychoanalysis was taken up as a profession, especially in the US, his theories were largely transformed into norms with which women had to comply. This meant that new neurotic conditions flourished, which stigmatized "women with psychological diagnoses that had their basis as much in the needs of medical and social conformity as in sexual difficulties."[70] In post-Second World War America, tropes such as "the frigid woman" and "the nymphomaniac" became popular labels of psychic imbalance as "psychoanalysis flourished as a far more normative profession than Freud had ever imagined."[71]

The Freudian "theory of the girl's anatomical deficiency" was one such essentialist view. This thesis included a view of woman as castrated, "leading to the female version of the Oedipus complex, which comprised penis envy, feelings of inferiority or self-hatred, and contempt for the mother."[72]

Feminist thinkers such as Simone de Beauvoir in her classic *The Second Sex* showed that woman had always been defined in relation to man, and challenged Freud's idea of gender relations. Betty Friedan and Kate Millett in America, Germaine Greer and Juliet Mitchell in Britain, among many others, pointed out the part Freud's psychoanalysis had played in women's oppression in the West.[73] For Millett, one of the main problems of Freud's theories was that it individualized the family dynamics and "undercut an engagement in sexual politics, the very possibility of women acting as the collectivity they in fact were."[74] Within the conservative iteration of psychoanalysis, resistance to stereotypes of motherhood or wifeliness was classified as neurosis and women who refused to conform were deemed crazy.

Phyllis Chesler published her seminal book *Women and Madness* in 1972, where she argued that definitions of mental illness were directly linked to conventional understandings of femininity and masculinity, and that any norm violation tended to be understood as madness. But as the 1970s progressed, the field of women's studies began to be established and there was a move by many feminist scholars to themselves train as psychoanalysts and psychologists. This meant that an increasing number of women populated the psychoanalytic field, and the profession gradually became less male-dominated.[75]

One of the feminist analysts was Juliet Mitchell, whose 1974 book *Psychoanalysis and Feminism* began to salvage psychoanalysis and highlight Freud's importance for the feminist project. In Europe Jacques Lacan's development of psychoanalysis was highly influential among feminists. In Lacan's interpretation, the phallus did not correspond to the literal penis, but to the symbolic order of civilization where the phallus was most valued. For the feminists following in his footsteps, "psychoanalytic thinking, which posited a dynamic psychic reality and no gendered essentials, was women's best hope of escaping a reduction to essentialist terms."[76]

Antipsychiatry and the Radical Schizophrenic

In conjunction with the feminist critique and redefinition of psychoanalysis grew a wider antipsychiatry movement, spearheaded by R.D. Laing in the UK. Together with Aaron Esterson, Laing conducted a study of women who had been hospitalized as chronic schizophrenics, which concluded that the cause of their illness was in their family situation and not in their biological makeup.[77] Laing's theories blossomed around the height of 1960s counterculture, and his stance on schizophrenia was that it was not a mental illness but "a mode of insight and prophecy."[78] In this framework psychosis was glorified as the route to spiritual and religious wisdom, much like the LSD trips popular at the time.

In 1965, to test their theories about schizophrenia, Laing and a group of antipsychiatrists started an experimental clinic at Kingsley Hall in East London.[79] Showalter points out that Laing's theories generally held that women were being unfairly institutionalized and that schizophrenia was partly caused by the role women had been given in a patriarchal society. When the clinic at Kingsley Hall opened, however, all of the doctors were men, and "the model patient was a woman."[80] In practice, women never obtained the status of doctor, which, no matter how much antipsychiatrists critiqued it, remained a position of great authority. Laing even had a "star schizophrenic," just like Charcot had his star hysterics. Mary Barnes, a 40-year-old catholic nurse, became, as Showalter puts it, Laing's Augustine.

Barnes had a long history of mental illness and had been hospitalized in other institutions for years before coming to Kingsley Hall. What set her apart from the institutionalized hysterics of the previous century was that she herself sought out Laing's treatment. She had read his influential book *The Divided Self* and concluded that his experimental methods were going to cure her. She also wrote her own narrative about her experiences at Kingsley Hall, in addition to establishing herself as a painter, with her artwork being displayed to the public on multiple occasions. Barnes became the face of the English antipsychiatry movement, even having a play written about her time at Laing's clinic.[81]

THE RISE OF PSYCHOPHARMACEUTICALS

As the cultural fascination with schizophrenia faded, the consumption of psychopharmaceuticals outside of the institution increased and became the new venue through which feminine coded madness expressed itself. This coincided with the gradual process of closing asylums in Europe and the United States, which was partly influenced by government cutbacks and anti-psychiatry movements, but whose primary instigator was the development of said psychopharmaceutical drugs.[82] In the US, this move began in 1955 with the widespread introduction of the antipsychotic drug chlorpromazine, commonly known as Thorazine, and was further enacted 10 years later with the introduction of the federal health care programs Medicare and Medicaid.[83]

The history of American psychiatry is often told as that of a professional field that in its early years was heavily influenced by psychoanalysis (and dominated by its restrictive gender roles), but sometime in the 1970s was taken over by neuroscience and an "objective" prescription of pills.[84] An important part of this was the development, and transformation of, the American Psychiatric Association's *Diagnostic and Statistical Manual of Mental Disorders* (DSM). The first edition was published in 1952 and was largely made up of psychoanalytical disorders that "assumed presenting symptoms, and, indeed, personality itself, to be the result of early life conflicts that were mapped onto the unconscious psychical apparatus for the remainder of life."[85] In the 1970s, however, a series of randomized clinical research studies revealed the benefits of biological psychiatry and psychopharmacology. In this new framework, "scientific findings laid bare neural pathways that exposed the inner workings of the mind."[86] The result was the creation of an "'objectifiable, biological' psychiatry that eschewed the role of early-life experience to identity formation and instead looked beneath these constructs to the level of the anatomic substrate."[87] And most importantly, the primary treatment for the biological mental disorders was psychopharmaceutical rather than psychoanalytical or psychodynamic.

This change was reflected in the third edition of the DSM, published in 1980 and significantly reworked under the leadership of Robert Spitzer. Previous to this edition psychiatrists often had different understandings of the same diagnosis and the aim was to create a reliable system with stable definitions of mental disorders. 25 committees, made up of scientifically inclined, anti-psychoanalytic, psychiatrists, were created to come up with detailed definitions of diagnoses. Each diagnosis included in the DSM-III came with a checklist of symptoms, and specific criteria for how many of these symptoms needed to be present for a diagnosis to be made.[88] With the new criteria, the American Psychiatric Association had created "a manual with a biomedical 'viability'."[89] The DSM-III and its subsequent editions have had an enormous impact on psychiatry worldwide, as it is the most widely used diagnostic manual globally, employed by psychiatrists almost everywhere to determine diagnoses.

As Appignanesi critically points out, two important driving forces behind the remaking of the DSM and the turn towards a biological psychiatry were pharmaceutical and insurance companies. "Big Pharma" requested standardization of disorders so as to be able to show medication's efficiency with particular demographics, and insurers wanted measurable symptoms/illnesses so as to regulate their payments.[90] When the DSM was imported to Europe and countries with public health care, the text was used by governments to decide which treatments to cover.

The DSM made psychiatry a quantifiable science, like other medicine, and removed the fuzziness of psychoanalysis and other psychotherapies. This was especially important for insurance companies and governments, where the set diagnoses of the DSM alongside its quantifiable talk therapy colleague—cognitive behavioral therapy (CBT)—gave those in charge of paying for treatments a range of measurable evidence of efficiency.[91] A cynical reading of this kind of treatment is that a prescription and ten sessions of CBT makes the patient ready for the labor market again.

Jonathan Michel Metzl has also critiqued the idea that the shift from psychotherapy to bio-psychiatry in mainstream treatments of mental illness left the biased psychoanalytical assumptions about gender and the family behind, letting the tangible "truth" of biology take its place. Metzl argues that the psychiatric discourse that claims to have displaced the gender roles of psychoanalysis via its reliance on an "objective" biology, in fact, maintains and reproduces these very roles. Through a detailed analysis of pop cultural representations of psychotropic drugs, he shows how medications and their cultural representations have worked in dynamic ways to influence the development of psychopharmacology itself. His study ranges from the release of the first "miracle cure for anxiety," Miltown, in the 1950s, via the tranquilizer craze of the 1960s and 70s with Valium at its center, to the ubiquitousness of Prozac in the 1990s.[92]

Throughout the development of psychopharmacology, the connection between femininity and mental dis-ease remained strong, despite the bio-psychiatrical promises of "objective" approaches that went beyond gender. The "'emotional' problems [that] could be cured simply by visiting a doctor, obtaining a prescription, and taking a pill" were primarily marketed as cures against female ailments, such as "a woman's frigidity, to a bride's uncertainty, to a wife's infidelity."[93] Metzl suggests that the anxieties surrounding mothers, and the accompanying framing of psychotropic drugs as the "saviors" of women who risked to reject traditional gender roles, was in reality a worry about the destabilization of traditional family norms. As the worries about traditions changed, so did the model patient for psychopharmaceuticals. In the 1950s it was the frigid or cheating wife who needed to be medicated, in the 1960s and 1970s it was the feminist who dared to question patriarchal institutions like marriage and essentialist male-female roles. In the 1990s and early 2000s, the workplace became the primary site for gender "struggles." Drugs like Prozac promised to keep the working woman upbeat and optimistic so that she could perform the tasks required by her particular line of work.[94]

Anorexia and Eating Disorders

Metzl's argument speaks, again, to the relation between the specific pathologizations of women and contemporary gender relations. Another set of diagnoses that have been highly feminized is anorexia and accompanying eating disorders. Susan Bordo has written significantly about their role in Western culture as diseases that primarily affect women and that arose as particularly prominent in the 1980s and 1990s.[95] Eating disorders might take their most visible form on the physical body, but they are firmly rooted in the mind, and thus belong to the "family" of psychopathologies. Bordo's analysis is rooted in Foucauldian theories of how power/knowledge structures come to discipline the body and psyche down to the level of influencing the process of subjectivation. In that vein she argues that "the escalation of eating disorders into a significant social phenomenon arises at the intersection of patriarchal culture and post-industrial capitalism."[96] Eating disorders, then, are strongly connected to the social and cultural context in which they are found. Bordo further argues that anorexia is not an individual expression of a pathology, but "a remarkably overdetermined *symptom* of some of the multifaceted and heterogeneous distresses of our age."[97]

Psychotherapist Susie Orbach argued in a similar vein, based on her own experience treating women with eating disorders, that anorexia is "a hunger strike, a protest against times which hold out the promise of independence and a life lived beyond the home while simultaneously demanding that women, as lovers, wives, mothers or carers, service the needs of others."[98] Orbach's book, *Hunger Strike: The Anorectic's Struggle as a Metaphor for Our Age,* was first published in 1986 and has since become a classic printed in multiple editions. In both Bordo's and Orbach's arguments, we see again how larger anxieties in society and culture are expressed in the pathologization of female mental health. They both also make the case for a feminist interpretation of self-starving as an act of protest, and thus they echo earlier feminist readings of mental dis-ease as a refusal of feminine conventions, such as those of fictional portrayals of Victorian madwomen and the rebellious schizophrenic. But crucially, the connections between eating disorders and feminist rebellion are not presented as conscious choices by the suffering individuals. Bordo directly states that "anorexia is not a philosophical attitude; it is a debilitating affliction," and remarks that "these pathologies of female protest … actually function as if in collusion with the cultural conditions that produced them."[99] This opens up for an understanding of mental illness diagnoses as affected and influenced by contemporary social mores without seeing the sociocultural connection as "proving" that the affliction is "made up" or only socially constructed. In other words, the fact that social structures are reflected in the popularity of a particular diagnosis does not take away from the suffering experienced by those who have received it.

Feminist Approaches to Psychopharmaceuticals

Feminist interpretations of medical diagnoses and treatments were prominent also in relation to the introduction of Prozac on the mainstream cultural and medical scene in the early 1990s, when narratives of women taking the drug were abundant. Judith Kegan Gardiner addresses feminist approaches to these narratives and to psychopharmacology in general in her influential essay "Can Ms. Prozac Talk Back? Feminism, Drugs, and Social Constructionism" from 1995. In it she reviews three of the most prominent contemporary books about Prozac, the first two written by medical professionals: Peter D. Kramer's *Listening to Prozac: A Psychiatrist Explores Antidepressant Drugs and the Remaking of the Self* (1993); Peter R. Breggin and Ginger Ross Breggin's *What Doctors Won't Tell You About Today's Most Controversial Drug* (1994); and writer Elizabeth Wurtzel's autobiography *Prozac Nation: Young and Depressed in America* (1994).

Writing at a time when feminist scholarship still held on firmly and unequivocally to the idea that women's depression was a result of patriarchy, Kegan Gardiner addresses the contradictory behavior she had encountered in personal meetings with other feminist scholars. The theoretical consensus seemed to be that there were no biological components to depression, only negative social circumstances. But Kegan Gardiner describes how she repeatedly met feminist scholars who held this critical position while simultaneously taking Prozac themselves to alleviate depressive symptoms. This led her to ask "what drugs like Prozac mean for women today and what the discourses about them say to and about American feminism."[100]

Kegan Gardiner's reading of the two physicians' texts shows how they exemplify contesting opinions of Prozac at the time. For Kramer, the drug works miracles in freeing women from traditional female roles, and he even calls it outright feminist and empowering.[101] Breggin and Breggin hold the almost opposite view, which Kegan Gardiner describes as similar to cultural feminism, extolling "women's traditional virtues, including maternal nurturance and empathy, and view[ing] women as endangered by the patriarchal violence of doctors and the drug industry."[102]

Wurtzel's autobiographical narrative, which Kegan Gardiner also reviews, instead recounts a firsthand experience of taking Prozac.[103] Wurtzel is a professional woman—a Harvard student and successful journalist who "portrays herself as the daughter of an abandoning father and an overinvolved mother."[104] She has a long history of depression and has had multiple therapists without results. Relief comes when she meets her first psychiatrist who prescribes her Prozac. The drug alleviates her symptoms and helps her recover from depression. Importantly, Wurtzel does not portray Prozac as a wonder drug that immediately cures, but sees it as a necessary tool in addition to therapy.[105] Autobiographical and fictional narratives like Wurtzel's were plentiful in the 1990s, all following similar trajectories of finding relief from the drug, then having it wear off and result in disappointment and regression, to finally end in a more or less balanced mental state.[106]

Are the "Ms Prozacs" in these narratives equivalent to the hysteric Augustine or the schizophrenic Mary Barnes? The fact that Wurtzel's book became a best seller and was turned into a feature film in 2001 suggests that "Ms Prozac"-narratives took hold in American culture. As such the young woman on anti-depressants can be seen as the embodiment of female madness in the late twentieth and early twenty-first century. Narratives like Wurtzel's, which assign positive attributes to anti-depressants, might seem to propagate a view that always deems drugs necessary in the treatment of depression. But paying attention to details, these stories also portray ambivalence about taking psychopharmaceuticals.

Here again then is the question that keeps resurfacing in the various analyses of femininely coded mental illness regarding its cause. Is female madness socially constructed or rooted in a biological and incontestable "truth"? If it is the former, is madness available as a radical tool to oppose power structures, as many feminist scholars of literary madness narratives have argued? And if it is the latter, do we have to give up on any attempt at viewing mental health as anything other than what the current biopsychiatric episteme holds to be true? What scholars like Bordo, Kegan Gardiner, Metzl, and Wilson suggest, is that there is an in-between where the complex entanglements of psyche and soma can be explored.[107] And as Appignanesi points out, "in a rampantly medicalized age, the classification of depression or borderline carries not stigma but the hope of cure."[108] Whereas in previous eras a diagnosis might have meant confinement, significant limitations to one's life, and rampant stigma, in the early twenty-first century, a diagnosis is in many places what will guarantee support and relief.

The discourses around diagnoses like depression, anxiety, bipolar disorder, and more that I examine in the rest of the book are in indirect dialogue with the history of female pathologizations of mental health explored in this chapter. I hope to have shown that there are clear connections between contemporary sociocultural discourses and popular mental illness diagnoses in that understanding of what is wrong with suffering women always takes shape in a larger cultural context that inevitably informs the articulation of dis-ease.

While women's sad experiences historically have been classified as pathologies leading to institutionalization and confinement, in the early twenty-first century, they tend to be medicalized within a biochemical discourse that reverts to (deinstitutionalized) psychotropic drugs and psychotherapy as solutions. In this way, the current pathologization of women's sad experiences takes place within a neoliberal framework that does not position them as abject and (completely) other, but instead renders them intelligible within a larger culture of self-help in which the individual is responsible for her own wellbeing.[109] In this framework, all ties between health and structures of inequality are severed, and any attempts at politicizing widespread ill health are thwarted. In the chapters to come I argue that this mode of thinking about mental health is dominant, but not all-encompassing in contemporary popular culture. Alongside the profitable vulnerability of the most mainstream representations of mental illness, there are several sites where ties between mental wellbeing and larger power structures are being made, most explicitly in *Teen Vogue* and among the sad girls on Instagram. In these spaces of sad girl culture, more radical understandings of feeling bad can be found, where both the suffering of those who struggle is acknowledged and critical analyses of the structural causes of diagnoses are spoken.

NOTES

1. Appignanesi, *Sad, mad and bad*; Chesler, *Women's madness*; Showalter, *The female malady*.
2. Chesler, *Women's madness*.
3. Wilson, *Psychosomatic: Feminism and the neurological body*.
4. Appignanesi, *Sad, mad and bad*; Showalter, *The female malady*.

5. Foucault, *Discipline and punish*.
6. Ibid; Foucault, *History of madness*.
7. Foucault, *The Birth of the Clinic*.
8. Showalter, *The female malady*, 8.
9. Ibid, 8.
10. Ibid, 8.
11. Ibid, 8.
12. Ibid, 8.
13. Appignanesi, *Sad, mad and bad*, 50.
14. Ibid, 50.
15. Showalter, *The female malady*, 10.
16. Showalter, *The female malady*, 8.
17. Showalter, *The female malady*, 38.
18. Appignanesi, *Sad, mad and bad*, 115.
19. Ibid, 126.
20. Showalter, *The female malady*, 10.
21. Ibid, 13.
22. Ibid, 14.
23. Gilbert and Gubar, *The madwoman in the attic*, 88.
24. Ibid, ix.
25. Caminero-Santangelo, *The madwoman can't speak*, 1.
26. Ibid.
27. Ibid, 132.
28. Didi-Huberman, *Invention of hysteria*, 6, emphasis in original.
29. Showalter, *The female malady*, 2.
30. Didi-Huberman, *Invention of hysteria*, 4.
31. Free and Brown, "Freeing the insane."
32. Didi-Huberman, *Invention of hysteria*.
33. Showalter, *The female malady*, 148, 167-168.
34. Didi-Huberman, *Invention of hysteria*, 68.
35. Ibid, 68, emphasis in original.
36. Ibid, 67, 68, emphasis in original.
37. Ibid, 69, emphasis in original.
38. Showalter, *The female malady*, 147.
39. Didi-Huberman, *Invention of hysteria*, 115.
40. Ibid, 115.
41. Showalter, *The female malady*, 148.
42. Didi-Huberman, *Invention of hysteria*, 32, emphasis in original.
43. Ibid, 32.
44. Ibid, 88-89.
45. Bourneville and Régnard, *Iconographie photographique de la Salpêtrière*.
46. Ibid, 157.

47. Showalter, *The female malady*, 154.
48. See Chesler, *Women's madness*; Showalter, *The female malady*; Showalter, *Hystories*.
49. Wilson, *Psychosomatic: Feminism and the neurological body*.
50. Ibid, 5.
51. Showalter, *The female malady*, 154.
52. Wilson, *Psychosomatic: Feminism and the neurological body*, 6.
53. Bourneville and Régnard, *Iconographie photographique de la Salpêtrière*, plate XIV.
54. Appignanesi, *Sad, mad and bad*, 152.
55. Ibid, 155; Showalter, *The female malady*, 156.
56. Showalter, *The female malady*, 156.
57. Ibid, 158.
58. Appignanesi, *Sad, mad and bad*, 160.
59. Foucault, *The history of sexuality*.
60. Appignanesi, *Sad, mad and bad*, 222.
61. Ibid, 223.
62. Showalter, *The female malady*, 155-158.
63. Didi-Huberman, *Invention of hysteria*, 157.
64. Showalter, *The female malady*, 204.
65. Ibid, 213.
66. Ibid, 213.
67. Appignanesi, *Sad, mad and bad*, 363.
68. Ibid, 285.
69. Ibid, 401.
70. Ibid, 227.
71. Ibid, 227.
72. Showalter, *The female malady*, 199.
73. Appignanesi, *Sad, mad and bad*, 418-419.
74. Ibid, 419.
75. Ibid, 422.
76. Ibid, 423.
77. Laing and Esterson, *Sanity, madness, and the family*.
78. Showalter, *The female malady*, 229.
79. Ibid, 230.
80. Ibid, 232.
81. Ibid, 232-236.
82. Appignanesi, *Sad, mad and bad*, 413.
83. Torrey, *Out of the shadows*, 8.
84. Metzl, *Prozac on the couch*, 1.
85. Ibid, 1.
86. Ibid, 1.

58   F. THELANDERSSON

87. Ibid, 2.
88. Appignanesi, *Sad, mad and bad*, 526-527.
89. Ibid, 528.
90. Ibid, 528-529.
91. Ibid, 529.
92. Metzl, *Prozac on the couch*, 72-73, 163-199.
93. Ibid, 72.
94. Ibid, 15.
95. Bordo, *Unbearable Weight*.
96. Ibid, 32.
97. Ibid, 141, italicization in original.
98. Appignanesi, *Sad, mad and bad*, 446; Orbach, *Hunger Strike*.
99. Bordo, *Unbearable Weight*, 150, 159.
100. Kegan Gardiner, "Can Ms. Prozac Talk Back?," 502.
101. Kramer, *Listening to prozac*.
102. Kegan Gardiner, "Can Ms. Prozac Talk Back?," 508-509; Breggin and Breggin, *Talking back to Prozac*.
103. Wurtzel, *Prozac nation*.
104. Kegan Gardiner, "Can Ms. Prozac Talk Back?," 509.
105. Ibid, 509.
106. Metzl, "Prozac and the pharmacokinetics of narrative form."
107. Bordo, *Unbearable Weight*; Kegan Gardiner, "Can Ms. Prozac Talk Back?;" Metzl, *Prozac on the couch*; Wilson, *Psychosomatic: Feminism and the neurological body*.
108. Appignanesi, *Sad, mad and bad*, 506.
109. Franssen, "The celebritization of self-care;" Johnson, "Managing Mr. Monk;" Rose, *Inventing our Selves*.

References

Appignanesi, Lisa. *Sad, Mad and Bad: Women and the Mind Doctors from 1800*. London: Virago Press, 2008.
Bordo, Susan. *Unbearable Weight: Feminism, Western Culture, and the Body*. Tenth anni. Berkeley, Los Angeles, London: University of California Press, 2003.
Bourneville, Désiré Magloire, and Paul-Marie-Léon Régnard. *Iconographie Photographique de La Salpêtrière*. Paris: Bureaux du Progrès médical/Delahaye and Lecrosnier, 1879.
Breggin, Peter R., and Ginger Ross Breggin. *Talking Back to Prozac: What Doctors Won't Tell You about Today's Most Controversial Drug*. New York: St. Martin's Press, 1994.
Caminero-Santangelo, Marta. *The Madwoman Can't Speak: Or Why Insanity Is Not Subversive*. Ithaca, New York: Cornell University Press, 1998.

Chesler, Phyllis. *Women's Madness: Misogyny or Mental Illness?* New York & London: St. Martin's Griffin, 2005.

Didi-Huberman, Georges. *Invention of Hysteria: Charcot and the Photographic Iconography of the Salpêtrière.* Cambridge, MA and London, England: The MIT Press, 2003.

Foucault, Michel. *Discipline and Punish.* New York: Random House LLC, 1977.

Foucault, Michel. *The History of Sexuality, Vol. 1. The Will to Knowledge. History of Sexuality.* New York & Toronto: Random House, 1978.

Foucault, Michel. *The Birth of the Clinic: An Archaeology of Medical Perception.* New York: Vintage, 1994.

Foucault, Michel. *History of Madness.* Vol. 1. Oxon, UK: Routledge, 2006.

Franssen, Gaston. "The Celebritization of Self-Care: The Celebrity Health Narrative of Demi Lovato and the Sickscape of Mental Illness." *European Journal of Cultural Studies* 23, no. 1 (2020): 89–111. https://doi.org/10.1177/1367549419861636.

Free, Elizabeth, and Theodore M. Brown. "Freeing the Insane." *American Journal of Public Health* 96, no. 10 (2006).

Gilbert, Sandra M., and Susan Gubar. *The Madwoman in the Attic: The Woman Writer and the Nineteenth-Century Literary Imagination.* 2nd ed. New Haven and London: Yale University Press, 2000.

Johnson, Davi A. "Managing Mr. Monk: Control and the Politics of Madness." *Critical Studies in Media Communication* 25, no. 1 (2008): 28–47. https://doi.org/10.1080/15295030701851130.

Kegan Gardiner, Judith. "Can Ms. Prozac Talk Back? Feminism, Drugs, and Social Constructionism." *Feminist Studies* 21, no. 3 (1995): 501–17.

Kramer, Peter D. *Listening to Prozac: A Psychiatrist Explores Antidepressant Drugs and the Remaking of the Self.* New York: Viking Penguin, 1993.

Laing, R.D., and Aaron Esterson. *Sanity, Madness, and the Family: Families of Schizophrenics.* Baltimore, MD: Penguin, 1970.

Metzl, Jonathan. "Prozac and the Pharmacokinetics of Narrative Form." *Signs: Journal of Women in Culture and Society* 27, no. 2 (2001): 347–80. https://doi.org/10.1017/CBO9781107415324.004.

Metzl, Jonathan. *Prozac on the Couch: Prescribing Gender in the Era of Wonder Drugs.* Durham and London: Duke University Press, 2003.

Mitchell, Juliet. *Psychoanalysis and Feminism: Freud, Reich, Laing and Women.* New York: Pantheon Books, 1974.

Orbach, Susie. *Hunger Strike: The Anorectic's Struggle as a Metaphor for Our Age.* London and New York: Routledge, 2005.

Rose, Nikolas. *Inventing Our Selves: Psychology, Power, and Personhood.* Cambridge, New York and Melbourne: Cambridge University Press, 1998.

Showalter, Elaine. *The Female Malady: Women, Madness, and English Culture, 1830-1980.* New York: Pantheon Books, 1985.

Showalter, Elaine. *Hystories: Hysterical Epidemics and Modern Culture.* New York: Columbia University Press, 1997.

Torrey, E. Fuller. *Out of the Shadows: Confronting America's Mental Illness Crisis.* New York: John Wiley & Sons, 1997.

Wilson, Elizabeth A. *Psychosomatic: Feminism and the Neurological Body.* Durham and London: Duke University Press, 2004.

Wurtzel, Elizabeth. *Prozac Nation: Young and Depressed in America.* New York: Houghton Mifflin, 1994.

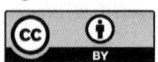

CHAPTER 3

Mental Health in Magazines: Relatability and Critique in *Cosmopolitan* and *Teen Vogue*

As instructive texts for how to live, women's magazines have been of interest to feminist scholars as reproducers of social norms and structures. The emergence of digital media has significantly weakened the hold of magazines on popular women's discourse, leading to declining revenues as advertisers and readers move to free online platforms.[1] But as publications with large corporations behind them, they are still worthy of study as representatives of traditional advice media that espouse scripts for how to approach mental health. This chapter thus looks at conversations around depression and anxiety in the online archives of *Cosmopolitan* (US) and *Teen Vogue*, based primarily on material published from 2008–2018. I examine the different orientations of these magazines when it comes to mental health by discussing their respective styles, tone, narratives, mode of address, and types of pedagogy and support around these issues.

Angela McRobbie's study of the girls' magazine *Jackie* was one of the first and most influential feminist analyses of this media genre.[2] McRobbie argues that publications in this genre "define and shape the woman's world, spanning every stage from early childhood to old age [where] the exact nature of the woman's role is spelt out in detail, according to her age and status."[3] One aspect of this guidance was the supportive function provided by these magazines, often in the form of advice columns where experts answered questions about everything from relationships to medical problems.[4]

© The Author(s) 2023

F. Thelandersson, *21st Century Media and Female Mental Health*,

https://doi.org/10.1007/978-3-031-16756-0_3

McRobbie describes how *Jackie* presents an ideal teenage girl whose interests and priorities go hand in hand with contemporary patriarchal and capitalist values. Other scholars have also identified magazines as key sites of cultural constructions of women, men, and gender relations.[5] Much of this research has contended that magazines convey damaging messages that propagate gender inequality and present a narrow feminine ideal centered on beauty, fashion, and romance. They have been read as promoting negative body ideals and leading to destructive dieting and plastic surgery,[6] as well as reproducing power hierarchies along the lines of class, race, and sexuality.[7]

As a postfeminist sensibility permeated media culture in the late 1990s and early 2000s, so magazines became important sites for postfeminist messaging. In simplified terms, at first this was expressed in the sense that feminist goals were seen as having already been achieved, so any larger social transformation along gender lines was unnecessary.[8] More recently a postfeminist sensibility has transformed into something more subtle, where feminism is acknowledged as important but reconceptualized in individual terms that emphasize choice, empowerment, and competition (see Chap. 1 for a more elaborate discussion of this).[9] This message is seen clearly in the world of magazines, where several outlets have declared their support of gender equality and incite their readers to become empowered and independent subjects.

Additionally, there is now a focus on "positive" images alongside the incitements to self-improvement. In her analysis of sex and relationship advice in *Glamour*, Rosalind Gill points out that women's magazines have always portrayed femininity as "contingent – requiring constant anxious attention, work and vigilance."[10] The advice of the current moment, however, is marked by an intensified self-surveillance that reaches into "entirely new spheres of life and intimate conduct," and focuses significantly on the psychological. The postfeminist subject is urged to change her attitude toward herself and become positive, rather than only change her physical appearance. For Gill, this is another way in which the psychic life of postfeminism expresses itself by restructuring its subject at the level of her subjectivity.[11]

One aspect that repeatedly comes up in the scholarly work on women's magazines is their contradictions, how they tend to present messages about being confident about your body alongside pages and pages of advertisements for how to diet and shape your body into submission. Gill notes that rather than seeing these contradictions as "the 'endpoint' of analysis of magazines," one might see it as "the contradictions doing ideo-logical work."[12] As an example Gill gives the "language of empowerment, equality and taking charge" which infuses the conversations around inti-mate entrepreneurship in *Glamour* magazine, but does so to promote tra-ditional rather than feminist ideals.[13] In this way the magazine avoids presenting a clearly traditional ideological message, and the presence of both feminist and anti-feminist ideas marks the outlet as distinctly postfeminist.

To examine the state of magazine discourse around mental health I chose *Cosmopolitan* because it is one of the oldest and most established women's magazines in the Anglophone world. It was also the most visited magazine website during the start of this project. *Teen Vogue* was then chosen as a second site because of its positioning as one of the strongest brands in contemporary girls' magazine culture in the mid-2010s. Even if it has not published print issues since December 2017, it lives on as a digi-tal magazine publisher and has branched out to "consumer experiences" like a biannual summit and a brand clothing line at Urban Outfitters.[14] The digital-only focus, the clothing line, and the summit makes *Teen Vogue* representative of how magazines respond to a "new media" land-scape where readers are consuming their content on digital rather than print platforms.

In terms of methodology, I used the search functions on the publica-tions' websites as well as their own tagging system. Overall, *Teen Vogue* had published more than twice the amount of articles on the topic of mental health and illness than *Cosmopolitan*.[15] The significantly higher number of pieces in *Teen Vogue* might suggest that mental health aware-ness is at the forefront of their brand, something I will discuss more below.

Cosmopolitan and *Teen Vogue's* online editions contained few traditional advice columns of the kind where experts answer readers' questions related to mental health. In fact, there was only one in each outlet throughout the primary decade studied here.[16] Even if there were barely any traditional advice columns, I consider the entire discourses of the magazines as dis-courses of advice, in the vein of "lifestyle media" which provide scripts for how to live.[17]

Next, I will discuss each publication and their dominant themes—their tone, mode of address, critical stance (and lack of one), and their approach to support—before doing a direct comparison of how both magazines covered the same celebrity events and science report.

COSMOPOLITAN

When Helen Gurly Brown rebranded *Cosmopolitan* to focus on sex and pleasure in 1965, the message stood in stark contrast to the women's magazines of the day that tended to focus on family and home economics. Brown successfully cemented the publication's "sex-centric brand of female empowerment"[18] and established its "fun, fearless female" ethos during her 32-year tenure.[19] According to David Machin and Joanna Thornborrow, who conducted a discourse analysis of 44 different national versions of *Cosmopolitan* from around the globe, the main discourse of the publication fosters the values of "independence, power and fun."[20] Machin and Thornborrow look at *Cosmopolitan's* coverage of sex and work, two topics that frequently take center stage in the magazine. They identify the contradictory ethos characteristic of women's magazines in this coverage, showing how *Cosmo* presents serious information about both sex and work, but then undercuts it by using a "tongue-in-cheek" tone which distances the article from both real sex and real work. The same light-hearted tone that marks the decades-old *Cosmopolitan* pieces about sex and careers can be found in the articles about mental health.

In this section I will discuss a few examples from the *Cosmo* archive that illustrates the dominant approach of the magazine to issues of mental health.

A Lighthearted and Distanced Tone

The lighthearted and tongue-in-cheek tone of *Cosmopolitan's* mental health coverage is on clear display in the outlet's many listicles. A listicle is an article where the majority of the content appears in the form of a list. The listicle became a popular type of internet "journalism," as it became an effective way to draw readers in by promising to condense almost any subject into easily digestible list form.[21] In this sense, the genre almost by default takes away the seriousness of a topic. The headline is an important part of this form, and looking at the titles of *Cosmo's* listicles reveals what kind of issues the magazine promises its readers to quickly deal with as well as who the assumed reader is. The earlier articles tend to adopt a mode of address that assumes you are interacting with someone else who is depressed or anxious, like "10 Things You Should Never Say To Someone With Depression" and its follow up "10 Things You Should Never Say to Someone With Anxiety."[22] Included in this category are also "13 Things

Not to Say to Someone Who Is Stressed Out," "17 Things to Never Say to a Girl With Borderline Personality Disorder," and "10 Things You Should Absolutely Not Say to a Woman With an Eating Disorder."[23] And even though the titles of these articles imply that the reader is the friend of someone who is suffering rather than the one suffering themselves, the content of the pieces is as much for someone with their own experience of mental illness as someone encountering it second hand, in that they traffic in a language of recognition. What these pieces have in common is the negative rhetorical approach of each list item, which states what NOT to say, before explaining why. For example, the first item on the list in "10 Things You Should Never Say To Someone With Depression" is simply "Everyone's depressed." The author, Anna Breslaw, explains "No, everyone *gets* depressed *sometimes*. It's normal to feel the repercussion of a bad day …. But diagnosed depression is like any other physical illness that requires medication. Like, you wouldn't say *"Everyone* has a thyroid problem."[24]

The later *Cosmo* listicles instead tend to appeal outright for identification in the headline, revealing a mode of address that assumes that the reader herself is suffering from these issues rather than asking for a friend. Examples include "16 Things Only Girls On Antidepressants Will Understand," "14 Struggles Only Girls With Anxiety Will Understand" and "12 Struggles Only Girls With Depression Will Understand."[25] Related to these are also "17 Dating Struggles Girls With Anxiety Understand" and "12 Dating Struggles Only Girls With ADHD Will Understand."[26] The first three, about antidepressants, anxiety, and depression, are all written by the same author and published a few days apart in May of 2016. As the headlines imply, these pieces invite the reader to join in recognition and agreement. These pieces were published during 2016 and 2017, later than most of the ones about what not to say to someone with a particular diagnosis, which might be a sign that the perception of the average *Cosmopolitan* reader has changed over time. Earlier in the decade, the editors at *Cosmopolitan* might have assumed that their readers did not themselves identify as having a particular diagnosis, but might be interested in reading about it if it was framed in terms of what to do if you encounter someone with a mental health issue. But later on, during 2016 and 2017, the average reader is assumed to herself be identifying as depressed, anxious, and on antidepressants.

In addition, the *Cosmopolitan* listicles tend to make full use of the layout to further set a lighthearted and tongue-in-cheek tone. Often each item on the list is accompanied by a GIF or an image to illustrate the point (this kind of illustration is present in 50% of the *Cosmo* listicles and only in one of the *Teen Vogue* ones). In "16 Things Only Girls On Antidepressants Will Understand," for example, a GIF of media personality Kimora Lee Simmons disapprovingly shaking her head accompanies item number four, "People asking you *why* you're on antidepressants is rude as hell," and a GIF of actress Molly Ringwald giving the middle finger in the film *The Breakfast Club* is displayed next to item number nine, "People who ask you if you've tried a "natural" solution, as if they're being *really* helpful."[27] The use of humorous visuals here serves to distance the reader from the seriousness of the topic discussed and presents a highly relatable self with which the reader can identify without feeling too much despair. This is similar to what Machin and Thornborrow describe in relation to the outlet's coverage of sex and work, where the tongue-in-cheek tone serves to create distance to real sex and real work.[28]

Common but Exceptional

One recurring angle presented in *Cosmopolitan* is that mental illness is both exceptional and common, as seen in the above quote about not telling someone who is depressed that "everyone's depressed." On the one hand, there is a strong focus on how having a certain diagnosis is NOT the same as being "a little sad" (which is articulated in several different ways, but with the purpose of differentiating the legitimate illness/diagnosis from a less serious and colloquial experience) and how it in this sense is exceptional (you are different than your friends who are just bummed out about a bad exam). Another example of this is "13 Things I Wish I Knew About Depression When I Was a Teenager" where number two on the list reads "Your friends might use the same words to describe how they feel, but they also might have no idea what you're going through."[29] In the accompanying bullet point the author laments clueless teenage friends who say they are depressed because of a bad grade, something that is not the same as suffering from clinical depression. Similarly, in "12 Struggles Only Girls With Depression Will Understand," item number three is simply "How loosely people use the word 'depressed.'" The author explains that there is a definitive difference between depression and sadness, stating that "Depression is chronic, while sadness is fleeting. Often times, depression isn't triggered by anything, while sadness usually is. So no, you're not sooo 'depressed' this season of *Game of Thrones* is over."[30] Here the hyperbolic tone ("you're not sooo 'depressed'") and the reference to popular culture also does the work of distancing the reader from the potential despair of depression by the use of humor.

On the other hand in this equation, depression is a common experience because it is just "like any other physical illness that requires medication"[31] and also you are not alone in having it, because the writer of the article shares your experience and so do all of the readers who clicked on it in recognition. This is also expressed in "13 Things I Wish I Knew About Depression When I Was a Teenager," where numbers three and four on the list are "That needing mental health help is the same as needing physical health help" and "There is no way you're the only kid at your school struggling with depression."[32]

In this framing, psychology and psychiatry are generally forces of good that are helping people while acknowledging a host of diseases that have just not previously been properly treated. Item number three on the list of what NOT to say to someone with depression exemplifies this. The statement that you are not supposed to say is "You don't need to be on medication—it's so overprescribed. Everyone's on drugs these days," which the author explains with:

> Yeah, because the medical health world is realizing that mental illnesses are just as serious as physical ones. It's easy to pass judgment on these kinds of medications because of a few college friends who managed to score recreational Adderall, but for every one of those, there are hundreds of people who have been pulled out of deep emotional and mental holes with the help of medication prescribed by good psychiatrists. You probably know some of them—you just don't know you do.[33]

Here the author first equates mental illness with physical illness, and in so doing reinforces a biomedical paradigm in which what is physiological is more important than "flimsy" psychological stuff. She then ascribes large potential and hope to medication and psychiatry by naming "hundreds of people who have been pulled out of deep emotional and mental holes." Within this framework, psychopharmaceuticals appear as a technology of hope which does the work of rescuing the subject from the despair of diagnosis.[34] The notion that "the medical health world is realizing that mental illnesses are just as serious as physical ones" also reinforces a positivist notion that mental illness diagnoses are out there in the world to be discovered, rather than discursive-material constructions bound up in particular socio-historical contexts.

The Relatable Self

Another theme that runs throughout the *Cosmo* pieces is the relatable self. In her study of a set of meme-based Tumblr blogs which portray everyday "girl" experiences, Akane Kanai identifies the production of "affectively relatable" online selves that touch upon difficult subjects but do so with self-deprecating humor that serves to defuse the seriousness of the problems.[35] The result is the production of a "relatable self" that never expresses too much vulnerability nor confidence. I contend that much of *Cosmopolitan*'s mental illness articles follow in this vein, and that their tongue-in-cheek tone serves the same purpose as the humor in Kanai's analysis—to produce a "relatable" self that is not too sad or too anxious. By packaging potentially heavy topics such as depression and anxiety in easy-to-digest listicles, illustrated by funny GIFs and packed with Internet slang such as OMG and STFU, one is disarming the topics of their seriousness and weight. This serves a double function—on the one hand, it lets *Cosmopolitan* cover serious topics without losing its "fun fearless female" voice, and in this sense, their writing on mental illness fits into the overall style and "feel" of its other pieces about things like sex and work. Like this, depression and anxiety also become tangible on the same level as these other topics (sex, beauty, work), where recognizing your own feelings in a funny listicle might make those feelings appear less overwhelming and more manageable. On the other hand, the comedic style in these pieces risks downplaying the seriousness of living with depression and anxiety.

Gill and Kanai identify the relatable self as one out of three "new modalities of feeling in neoliberalism," alongside "the imperative to confidence" and "the promotion of 'boldness' as a value in itself."[36] They describe an interesting interplay between negotiating incitements to confidence and the discussion of problems faced in the everyday of late capitalism in the blogs Kanai analyzes. They write:

> In directing lighthearted humor against the self, the blogs attempt to walk the line between traditional affective regulations that mandate girls and women apologize for their presence, please others, and take up less emotional space; and contemporary demands to singlehandedly demonstrate confident, positive selfhood in relation to the degrading conditions of contemporary capitalism.[37]

The role of humor here is to defuse the notion that one is overly impacted by "the degrading conditions of contemporary capitalism." A similar negotiation is happening in the *Cosmopolitan* listicles about mental illness, where the pains of living with an issue becomes intelligible as a common, and thus manageable, feature of contemporary life. One specific way this is being done is in the use of the word "basically" in the listicle "16 Things Only Girls On Antidepressants Will Understand." Number 2 on the list reads:

> Your body is basically a science experiment until you find the right meds. It's *so* rare to initially be prescribed the medication that's right for you, so you have to try lots of different meds out. But when you find that perfect combination of meds, you realize it was probably worth it.[38]

The phrase "your body is basically a science experiment" manages to describe an unpleasant situation in a slightly detached way, primarily by adding "basically" to the sentence, which disarms it of its seriousness. By emphasizing how common it is to have to try out several different medications before finding the right one, the listicle manages to normalize the potentially terrifying experience of being a "science experiment" and assure the reader who might be in the middle of that process to keep at it because it will be worth it in the end.

Comparing this to Kanai's blogs, where an expression and acknowledgment of problems is done in a humorous way so as to appear relatable and not "too much" to other bloggers and to third parties who might encounter them, the *Cosmopolitan* listicle here performs this relatability primarily to readers who are themselves going through the experience and might need reassurance that it is not as bad as it seems. By folding a distressing experience (trying out different drugs) into a medical framework in which it is just business as usual, *Cosmopolitan* here assures the reader that this potentially scary phase of managing a depression is common and reasonable. This approach might minimize the unpleasantness and difficulty of the process by providing some reassurance to readers for whom trivializing what they are going through can be a way of making it more manageable. By managing one's mental health issues like this, one might gain temporary personal relief, but any discussion of broader systems and possibilities is left untouched.

Firsthand Narratives of Suffering, Diagnosis, and Redemption

There are some *Cosmo* pieces that take a more serious tone, primarily those that present firsthand accounts of a certain illness that often include a narrative arc of suffering, diagnosis, and redemption. These are similar to what Lisa Blackman calls the victim-to-victor narrative found in anti-stigma campaigns, where the protagonist starts out by suffering, then receives a diagnosis, and is finally salvaged by the help of medication and therapy.[39] These kinds of narratives tend to construct psychiatry as a technology of hope, whereby the subject enters into successful recovery after having agreed to the diagnosis and treatment provided by professional experts. The personal stories in *Cosmopolitan* largely follow this script, although it is not always psychiatry that appears as the savior. In a piece titled "Why I Turn to YouTube When My Anxiety Gets Out of Control," author Kerry Justich shares her ways of coping with generalized anxiety disorder. Describing a recent panic attack caused by a cancellation of subway trains, after unsuccessfully having tried to reach her mother on the phone, Justich went home and opened up YouTube, where her "favorite family of vloggers" soothed her anxiety. Like in most personal stories published by *Cosmo*, Justich gives the reader the back story of her diagnosis—her parents divorced when she was 14, and since then she has tried to keep strict routines in her life, if these are not followed or something goes awry, she experiences severe anxiety. Justich describes the severity of it as follows: "My anxiety paralyzes me. It overwhelms my brain and body, forcing me to shut down. Everything I do, I second-guess. Everything I say, I quickly question. And everyone I know I fear might someday disappear from my life."[40] She then recounts how this anxiety came to a head during her senior year of high school, which is when she saw a therapist and psychologist and was diagnosed with generalized anxiety disorder. Interestingly, this professional did not suggest medication, only "meditation, counting, working out, writing, and using an ocean waves sound app," which goes against critical narratives that assume medication is always the first route suggested by psychological professionals. For Justich, however, none of the suggested methods were successfully able to quiet her mind. She explains that:

> In those moments, I crave human interaction, but when I am in an unsteady state of mind, I feel like I can't rely on my friends or family to fulfill those needs. YouTube is the one thing that could turn off my over-processing mind.[41]

In her analysis of the cultural production of female psychopathology in women's magazines, Lisa Blackman draws on Arlie Russell Hochschild's study of women's advice books published from the 1970s up through the early 1990s.[42] Hochschild compares earlier books which adopt a patriarchal view of the family, in which the woman is assumed to be unequal to her husband, with later books that adopt a (somewhat) feminist conception of family and intimate relationships, where husband and wife are seen to be equals. For Hochschild, the earlier, patriarchal pieces reflect more "warmth" than the more modern publications, which "call for more open and more equal communication, but ... propose 'cooler' emotional strategies with which to engage those equal bonds."[43] This reflects a "cultural cooling" in which the gains of second-wave feminism have mixed with the goals of capitalism, resulting in "a commercial spirit of intimate life," where "part of the *content* of the spirit of capitalism is being *displaced* onto intimate life."[44] Part of this commercialization of intimate life is the idealization of a self that is "well defended against getting hurt,"[45] Hochschild explains:

> The heroic acts a self can perform, in this view, are to detach, to leave and to depend and need less. The emotion work that matters is control of the feelings of fear, vulnerability and the desire to be comforted. The ideal self doesn't need much, and what it does need it can get for itself.[46]

Blackman picks up on Hochschild's "no-needs modern woman" and identifies her in the women's magazines of the early 21st century, where she appears as someone who "is the primary force in her own life and who is able to work on herself, through particular techniques of self-production, such that she can get by with relatively little support from others – particularly men."[47] Here, traditionally masculine "feeling rules" have been displaced on feminine intimate relationships, and women are urged to be more cool and detached in close relations.

The emotion the no-needs woman fears the most is "the desire to be taken care of, to be safe and warm, which is embodied in a fear of being dependent on another, even one's therapist."[48] For Blackman and Hochschild, the emotional needs that this feminine subject inevitably has, despite not wanting to have them, then become relegated to discourses of self-help (such as advice books or magazines) and professionalized discourses of therapy and counseling. Most importantly, they are shifted away from the intimate relationship or close family and friends to professionalized discourses. Turning back to the *Cosmopolitan* article from 2015, when Justich describes the worst moments of her anxiety, she says that she craves human interaction, but "when I am in an unsteady state of mind, I feel like I can't rely on my friends or family to fulfill those needs" and instead she turns to YouTube which is "the one thing that could turn off my over-processing mind." So here Justich goes against the "no needs modern woman" in the sense that she acknowledges that she longs for human interaction, but she then immediately disavows that real human interaction will be able to give her what she *actually* needs. In so doing she seems to construct human interaction as too messy and complicated (and perhaps requiring too much of reciprocated action), whereas watching human interaction on YouTube via her favorite vlogger family (Justich links to the SACCONEJOLYs, an Irish family with four small children who posts new videos about their life every day) provides her with the simpler, detached, and mediated experience of human interaction.[49]

In the last paragraph of the article Justich elaborates on her current relation to therapy and psychological professionals, saying that she has been able to depend on her therapist less now that she has YouTube. She says that she could use the therapist's help sometimes, but:

> I feel empowered to know I've made it so long on my own. Anxiety is something that I'll never live without, but knowing that relief is a literal click away provides me a little bit of peace in my otherwise chaotic mind.[50]

Here Justich exemplifies a hyper independence from not only family and friends, but also the professionals that should supposedly be there to help her. So instead of displacing the care from family and friends to a professional discourse, like Blackman and Hochschild describe in their analyses, here we have someone who has gone a step further and has managed to make it also without those professionals. And although this might be seen as resistance to the dominance of the psy-sciences and psychology professionals in managing mental health, it can also be read as a response to a nonfunctioning support system, say the failure of the mental health care system in the United States. And instead of requiring reforms to a broken system, or turning to one's family, *Cosmopolitan* is here encouraging you to self-medicate with digital media.

Additionally, by saying that she feels "empowered" for having survived without anyone else for so long she also invokes the language of popular feminism,[51] suggesting that she has gained something on a political level, although what she seems to have overcome here is only the dependence on others.

Definitions and Diagnoses

One last thing to note about *Cosmo's* coverage is the presence of specific definitions of what it means to be depressed, anxious, or in other mental distress. I ask about these with Blackman's discussion of the production of female psychopathology in women's magazines in mind. Here she urges scholars to examine "how the arena of relationships is made intelligible and what concepts allow the distinctions between the normal and the pathological to be thought."[52] One way to ask that question in relation to my empirical material is to ask if and how definitions of particular ailments are given. Is it assumed that the reader already knows what it entails to suffer from depression? What definitional work is happening and what stakes and boundaries are being laid out?

The early *Cosmo* articles tend to describe depression and anxiety more in general terms of "feeling bad" rather than mention specific diagnoses by name (even if they have been tagged with them), and the solutions presented tend to be focused on self-help techniques instead of psychiatric medications and therapy. The first and only article from 2009, for example, is titled "How to Beat the Winter Blues" and does mention the existence of the diagnosis Seasonal Affective Disorder (SAD) but suggests getting active physically and socially, watching your carbs, going on a mini-vacation, having sex, and "consider light therapy" as solutions without bringing up therapists or drugs.[53] This goes on until 2013, when depression as clinical illness starts popping up in the *Cosmo* pieces.[54] From 2014 and onward the majority of the articles in *Cosmo* feature discussion of specific diagnoses and mental health and illness appear as obvious aspects of contemporary life. For example, an article from 2015 titled "This Mom's Powerful Selfie Proves There's No Shame in Taking Anxiety Medication" features a viral Facebook post of a woman holding up prescriptions for antidepressant and anxiety medications in a selfie and stating in the caption that she was unashamed to be taking them.[55] The post led to multiple other women responding with their own stories of taking psychiatric medications under the hashtag #MedicatedAndMighty, something the *Cosmo* writer comments as follows: "I am a very anxious lady and I am loving this. Cheers to Jones, all these other women, and to reminding the world that needing medication isn't anything other than taking a step toward being healthy."

Next I will discuss the dominant themes in *Teen Vogue* and their generally serious approach to issues of mental health before providing a direct comparison of how the two outlets covered the same events.

TEEN VOGUE

Teen Vogue emerged in 2003 as an offshoot of the fashion magazine *Vogue* at the same time as other large magazines aimed at adults published their own teen versions, like *Elle Girl* (2001-2006), *CosmoGirl!* (1999-2008), and *Teen People* (1998-2006). During the first 13 years of its existence it published pieces typical for publications aimed at teenage girls, but it was significantly rebranded in 2016 when 29-year old, African-American, Elaine Welteroth took over as editor in chief.[56] Under Welteroth's leadership the magazine began publishing "more overtly political, and often feminist, articles" alongside traditional teen magazine fare like fashion and relationships.[57] One piece in particular put *Teen Vogue* on the map as serious in its political critique. In December 2016, shortly after the general election that made Donald Trump president, Lauren Duca published an article titled "Donald Trump Is Gaslighting America," which suggested that the president-elect was engaging in psychological manipulation of the American people.[58] The article spread quickly online and in the mainstream press, leading to much commentary about the surprising critical sharpness of the teen magazine. *Teen Vogue* has continued in this spirit since, publishing stories about political issues ranging from reproductive rights to Black Lives Matter.[59] At the time of writing, the footer on their website reads: "The young person's guide to conquering (and saving) the world. *Teen Vogue* covers the latest in celebrity news, politics, fashion, beauty, wellness, lifestyle, and entertainment."[60] In this way, attention to politics and critical thinking is folded into the *Teen Vogue* brand alongside more "shallow" topics like celebrities, fashion, and makeup. The publication was even hailed as a "rallying point of resistance" in Trump-era America, presumably succeeding in their mission.[61]

Feminist media scholars Natalie Coulter and Kristine Moruzi have analyzed *Teen Vogue's* position as a political outlet for girls by positioning it in relation to the Victorian girls' magazine *Girl's Realm* (1898–1914), which was known for its engagement with contemporary issues related to women's rights, such as women's suffrage. By making this historical comparison Coulter and Moruzi show that *Teen Vogue* does not exist in a presentist vacuum, but is part of a longer history of conceptualizing "the female reader as engaged with the social and cultural politics of their respective eras."[62] They argue that the ideal girl defined by *Teen Vogue* is someone who "has a political conscious that is explicitly labelled as 'woke.'"[63] "Woke" or "wokeness" has its recent legacy in the Black Lives Matter movement which popularized the term.[64] It often indicates a "critical consciousness of intersecting systems of oppression" that acknowledges the "oppression that exists in individual and collective experiences."[65] Coulter and Moruzi point out that the term changes in different circumstances and that *Teen Vogue* does not explicitly define what it means by "wokeness," but that Welteroth's use of the concept "implies that the magazine is articulating an awareness of social issues and the ways that systematic oppressions intersect."[66] They go on to state that part of the magazine's "wokeness" is that it "resists much of the familiar postfeminist narratives of empowerment and the aspirational fantasies of personal improvement ... that have been endemic in girls' print culture in the early twenty-first century."[67]

This ethos of "wokeness" is reflected also in the publication's coverage of mental illness when connections between mental health and systemic oppression are made (seen for example in a piece that connects depression and suicide rates among transgender kids with stigma and hostility against them or in an article about how racial discrimination causes stress in those who experience it).[68] This happens in 6% of all *Teen Vogue's* articles, which is not an overwhelming amount of times, but far more often than *Cosmopolitan* which only connects mental distress with structural inequalities in 1.5% of their pieces.

What stands out with *Teen Vogue's* mental health coverage is that it significantly increases in 2016, from having been in the single digits up until 2014, it increases to 23 pieces during 2015 but then significantly jumps to 137 articles during 2016. This increase in coverage might be a sign that articles relating to mental health fit well into the publication's updated and "woke" brand.

Providing Critical Context

The overall tone in *Teen Vogue* tended to be straightforward, earnest, and serious. One way this was expressed was in the kind of topics covered in their general interest category, which featured both more expected subjects like a story about how telepsychiatry lets therapists treat you via digital tools like Skype and FaceTime and more politically inflected stories like a hospital getting sued for discrimination after a transgender teen died by suicide after having been treated there.[69]

Taking a closer look at one of the stories in this category reveals the serious tone and critical stance adopted by the publication. In January

2017 *Teen Vogue* wrote about the fate of a black teenager, Bresha Meadows, who was accused of killing her father after she and her family endured years of abuse by him. The outlet reports that Meadows was transferred from the juvenile jail she had been staying in for 175 days to a mental health treatment facility to receive an evaluation. The author of the piece points out that "despite the change, Bresha will not be free to come and go from the treatment facility."[70] The support group that had formed around the hashtag #FreeBresha is then mentioned, as is the day of action taken to urge the judge to release Meadows from juvenile detention. Here *Teen Vogue* cites research that shows the inefficiency of such confinement not only by referring to the activist group, but also citing and linking to a report from the Justice Policy Institute that shows how "incarcerating young people does little to help them in the long run, instead increasing their chances of returning to jail or prison in the future."[71] The *Teen Vogue* writer, Brittany McNamara, then points out that the #FreeBresha group called attention to another important issue: "survivors of domestic abuse being punished." She cites research from the "Women in Prison Project of the Correctional Association of New York" which shows that "67% of women accused of killing someone close to them had been abused by that person" and that "of all the state's inmates in for any charge, 75% had experienced severe physical domestic violence."[72] This leads McNamara to state that "all too often, survivors of domestic violence are punished for their survival," before citing the official statement from the #FreeBresha group about why the teenager should be freed while awaiting trial. In many ways this is traditional reporting of a story like this—giving the reader the backstory of what had previously happened to Meadows in addition to describing the latest developments in the case. But McNamara adds a critical perspective to the story by referring to research both about the inefficiency of the juvenile jail system and the high levels of domestic violence victims among incarcerated women, making it not only a story about a singular teenage girl's tragic fate, but also about the larger problem of women who stand up to their abusers being punished by the legal system. In this way the outlet lives up to its ethos of wokeness. Additionally, by tagging this and similar stories with "mental health" and other relevant tags, it shows up among other, more personal and individual-focused pieces, and the reader learns to include also such structural issues in the scope of mental health.

Seriousness in Favor of Distanced Relatability

While *Cosmo* tends to have a tongue-in-cheek tone that presents issues in relatable ways without getting too threatening or uncomfortable, the tone in the *Teen Vogue* pieces is instead marked by a seriousness that treats mental illness in a straightforward and earnest way. This is seen in how different the listicles look in each outlet. *Teen Vogue* had fewer articles in this genre on the whole than *Cosmo* (8% versus 15%) and their listicles tended to maintain the somber tone of the outlet at large. This is seen in a few key differences in the layout of the listicles in the two outlets. The first of these is the introductory paragraph that *Teen Vogue* includes in all of their listicles, which presents the issue at hand and gives some context. An example of this kind of introduction is the following, which accompanies the piece "26 Date Ideas for Your Anxious Partner":

> Anxiety can often make dating a challenge—unfamiliar people and environments might heighten the mental and physical symptoms someone with anxiety faces. This can make it difficult to plan a first date, or even an outing with a long-term significant other.[73]

This gives the reader a framework for why folks with anxiety might need specific dating ideas, and what those ideas might look like. 100% of the *Teen Vogue* listicles include an introduction in this vein, compared to only 34% of the *Cosmo* listicles, which often jump straight into the list of relatable points. Another marked difference between the layout of listicles in the two outlets is the use of GIFs or humorous illustrations to accompany items on the list. Only 1 of *Teen Vogue's* listicles contained GIFs and comedic images, whereas 50% of *Cosmo's* listicles did the same. This contributes to an overall more serious tone in *Teen Vogue* and underscores the more relatable and easygoing approach taken by *Cosmo*. The presence of illustrations like these in *Cosmo* contributes to the more lighthearted tone of that publication and the lack of them in *Teen Vogue* in comparison contributes to its more earnest tone.

The above article is also an example of *Teen Vogue* collaborating with the website *The Mighty*, which is a media platform and digital community focused on connecting people facing health challenges and disabilities.[74] The 26 date ideas presented in the listicle at hand are pooled from *The Mighty* community members who themselves suffer from anxiety and have contributed what an ideal date looks like for them. *Teen Vogue* has a few similar pieces that are collaborations with the online therapy service Talkspace, while *Cosmo* does not have any similar collaborations.

This seriousness is also reflected in the topics of the listicles themselves. Within this category on the site one can, for example, find one titled "11 Things You Can Do To Help Black Lives Matter End Police Violence," which manages to both explain the importance of mental health in the Black Lives Matter movement (number eight on the list is "Advocate for mental health intervention" and explains how victims of police brutality often have mental health issues) and situate political causes like these in the context of mental health by tagging the article mental health and thus showing it to readers who are browsing those topics.[75] This is again a way in which the magazine lives up to its "wokeness."

Another example is the piece "11 Things You Can Do to Avoid Self-Harm" which is written by Vijayta Szpitalak, who is introduced as a "Columbia University trained licensed mental health counselor with a practice in New York since 2010."[76] This is an example of *Teen Vogue* employing experts in their mental health coverage, something they do in 14% of their articles (compared to 9% of *Cosmo's* pieces). Taking a closer look at how this piece is structured reveals how *Teen Vogue* tends to address its readers.

The article starts with a trigger warning stating that it "contains detailed information about self-harm in the form of cutting and may be disturbing for some readers." The text then begins by addressing the reader directly, stating "chances are you or someone you know cuts themselves" before mentioning two celebrities who have been open about their cutting (Angelina Jolie and Demi Lovato). Szpitalak then introduces self-harm and cutting by stating first how common it is (citing research that shows 46% of high school students in the US having engaged with it at some point) and then explaining what self-harm actually is. This bare-bones definition reads: "a maladaptive method of coping that involves non-suicidal self-infliction of pain in the form of cutting, using anything from fingernails to razor blades, burning themselves, or preventing previous wounds from healing."[77] This is an example of *Teen Vogue* not only mentioning clinical diagnoses but also providing definitions from experts or professional sources of how certain mental illness issues are medically defined, which I discuss more below.

Szpitalak then describes how there are a number of reasons why people might engage in self-harming behavior before including a quote from a (child and adolescent) psychiatrist about possible reasons for cutting. And then she addresses the reader directly again: "It's important to first realize that cutting doesn't actually solve any problems, and isn't an effective method of coping for the long-term," before referencing research that has found a connection between self-harm and suicide attempts. It is not until after five opening paragraphs that the listicle itself is introduced with the following statement: "If you cut, it is possible to stop. The key is replacing the behavior with a healthy coping mechanism. It takes effort, love, and patience, but it can be done. As a starter, you can do the following." The list then reads as follows: "Identify triggers; Identify emotions; Tell someone; Seek professional help; Try a less severe form; Write your future self letters; Delay cutting; Consider Dialectical Behavior Therapy; Cultivate mindfulness; Feel a release; Stay positive."[78] There is a seriousness and weight given to the issue of self-harm here, which is treated like an (almost) life and death matter. With this piece *Teen Vogue* shows that it takes the issue of self-harm and its high prevalence among high school students very seriously, and in so doing it also encourages its readers to take their own and their peers' mental health seriously.

Compare this to *Cosmo*, who only mentions self-harm in three of their articles and when the issue appears it is only indirectly: It is mentioned briefly in relation to Demi Lovato; in a study about the antidepressant drug Paxil; and in one personal story/firsthand account where a writer describes writing publicly about her mental illness on social media as a form of self-harm.[79] In other words, Cosmo does not give the same weight to the issue of self-harm as *Teen Vogue* does. Perhaps this is because self-harm is an issue often associated with a demographic that is younger than *Cosmopolitan*'s target audience, or because it is hard to write about an issue like this while maintaining a distanced and lighthearted tone. Nevertheless, the coverage of self-harm in *Teen Vogue* and its absence in *Cosmo* is another example of the different orientations of each magazine.

Definitions and Diagnoses

When it comes to the presence of definitions of depression, anxiety, and other mental states, the changes over time in *Teen Vogue* are similar to *Cosmopolitan*, but more in the sense that there are few pieces published at all related to depression and anxiety up until 2015. From the second half of that year and onwards, almost all of the *Teen Vogue* pieces mention clinical diagnoses and biomedical treatments.[80] Again, this seems to suggest that the medical discourses around mental health became more mainstream and were assumed to be widely known from 2015 onward.

In *Teen Vogue* the definitional work is at times very explicit, in that they not only mention a clinical diagnosis but also provide lists of symptoms and other facts about the diagnosis at hand.[81] An example of this, in addition to the one above about self-harm, is an article about pop group One Direction canceling a concert because one of their members had an anxiety attack. Here the magazine explains that "anxiety disorders affect millions of people, and panic attack symptoms can range from shortness of breath, elevated heart rate, and even a choking feeling."[82] In the sentence, the phrase "millions of people" links to a page on the Anxiety and Depression Association of America's (ADAA) website with facts and statistics about anxiety and depression, which also includes links to information sites about various specific diagnoses, such as Generalized Anxiety Disorder, Social Anxiety Disorder, and Major Depressive Disorder.[83] By providing their readers with the symptoms of a panic attack and by linking to a website aligned with the medical establishment, *Teen Vogue* adopts a sort of pedagogical approach that assumes the reader might not know exactly what constitutes a panic attack, but might benefit from medical definitions that also include information on how to treat one.

Providing Support

What also marked *Teen Vogue's* approach to mental health was a dedication to providing support to its readers, which is shown clearly in their coverage of the Netflix series *13 Reasons Why*. The show, based on the 2007 young adult novel by Jay Asher, premiered on the streaming service March 31, 2017 and received widespread attention due to its handling of teenage suicide and mental illness. The story follows the aftermath of 17-year-old Hannah Baker's suicide, and the unraveling of the box of cassette tapes she recorded leading up to her death, in which she reveals why she choose to end her life. Baker recorded 13 tapes for 13 different people who she claims are responsible for her suicide, and throughout the first season, the viewer gets to follow her surviving friend Clay Baker as he goes through the tapes, featuring some tough scenes of sexual assault and bullying. The series quickly became popular among teenagers and young adults, but received criticism for glorifying suicide and risked spreading copycat behavior and self-harm among vulnerable groups.[84]

Teen Vogue published an op-ed on the day of the show's release, in which a suicide prevention advocate explains what is missing from the show. In the piece, MollyKate Cline says that "the audience is shown what *not* to do without examples of what they actually should do."[85] She points specifically to how Baker is never seen successfully reaching out for help to her peers or the adults in her life and that the show fails to mention depression or other mental health issues, which are common backdrops to suicide. Cline also points to the high numbers of suicide among teenagers in the US (it is the "second leading cause of death for ages 10–24, with 5,240 attempts per day from kids grades 7–12"), stating that the best way you can get help if you are being bullied or feeling suicidal is to tell someone, something she had hoped the show "would focus on instead of a dramatic story line over getting revenge for those 13 people."[86]

In 2017 *Teen Vogue* published 16 articles about *13 Reasons Why* and the controversy surrounding it (*Cosmo* did not cover the show at all). Looking at the content of these pieces, the publication appears concerned to provide its readers with nuanced and responsible coverage of a life and death topic. Among the articles is a set of quotes from teenagers themselves about the show (motivated by the fact that "dozens of articles have been written by adults, but fewer have shown the opinions of actual high school students") that also features input from a psychiatry professor;[87] a collection of resources for getting help if you have been experiencing depression or suicidal ideation after watching the show;[88] and an interview with suicide attempt survivors about the suicide scene in the series (which was heavily criticized as overly graphic and was deleted from the first season by Netflix in July 2019).[89] All of the articles contain some version of the following phrase at the end: "If you or someone you know is contemplating suicide, call the National Suicide Prevention Hotline at 1-800-273-8255 or text Crisis Text Line at 741-741." *Teen Vogue* seems to think about their readers' needs for support in relation to the show, and positions itself as a provider of that support.

The frequency with which *Teen Vogue* includes numbers to hotlines or links to other resources for those in distress is significant because it contributes to the overall serious tone of the publication when it comes to issues of mental health. In *Teen Vogue* 22% of articles include the phone number for the National Suicide Prevention Hotline (or equivalents like the Crisis Text Line and the National Eating Disorders Association Helpline) or links to sites with further resources (like the website of the phone hotlines or organizations like the Trevor Project, which is focused on helping LGBTQ-youth). This is compared to 10% of *Cosmo* articles featuring similar resources.

Interesting to note in *Teen Vogue*'s coverage of *13 Reasons Why* and of suicide in general, is their use of the phrase "died by suicide" instead of the commonly used "committed suicide." The former phrase is preferred by mental health advocates, as it removes culpability from the person who has lost their life and opens up for discussions of the disease or disorder they were suffering.[90] By employing the language of mental health advocates, the magazine consciously aligns itself with an anti-stigma/awareness discourse and acknowledges their own role as participants in the public discourse around mental health, including a recognition of the role of language in shaping this discourse.

This is seen clearly in their repeated mention of fighting stigma and on the value of speaking out about mental illness as an important step toward normalizing mental health issues. In their reporting about celebrities speaking out about mental health issues, for example, they tend to point out the inherent good of talking about it. In an article about an open letter written by Lady Gaga for the Born This Way Foundation's website (a foundation that seeks to "support the mental and emotional wellness of young people by putting their needs, ideas, and voices first") about living with PTSD, the writer recounts how Gaga shares that she is going to therapy and is taking medication, but feels that "the most inexpensive and perhaps the best medicine in the world is words" which is why she is speaking up. The *Teen Vogue* writer, Brittney McNamara, agrees and ends the article with the following statement:

> Lady Gaga is right. Keeping mental illness a secret gives power to the stigma that surrounds it and prevents so many people from accessing treatment. The more we talk about these things, the more people will realize they can—and should—get help. We're so glad she's been able to seek therapy, and we hope she inspires anyone in a similar position to do the same.[91]

The tone here is straightforward and earnest. McNamara seems happy for Lady Gaga and confirms the artist's belief in the power of words for fighting stigma and shame surrounding mental illness, confirming a logic underlying most celebrity confessions of mental illness, something I discuss further in Chap. 4.

Teen Vogue kept the trend of providing support to its readers during the COVID-19 pandemic, with a dedicated hub on their website titled "Days

Derailed: The Coronavirus Crisis."[92] Here readers could find a collection of articles about COVID-19 and the global health crisis that has emerged in the wake of the virus. The topics covered include what we know about the virus, advice for dating during a pandemic, how to overcome coronavirus anxiety, and what to do if you are quarantined with an abuser.[93] Alongside these pieces about the private and the personal was also an op-ed titled "The Coronavirus Pandemic Demonstrates the Failures of Capitalism" and a piece detailing the disproportionate impact of COVID-19 on the Black community.[94] Like this the readers who go to *Teen Vogue* for support in a time of crisis cannot avoid getting informed also about how the unequal distribution of wealth and institutionalized racism exacerbates the problems of the pandemic.

For the remaining part of this chapter, I will discuss how the two magazines covered the same celebrity events and the same study of a popular antidepressant. This comparison reveals the different orientations of the two publications.

DIFFERENT APPROACHES TO CELEBRITY REPORTING

When it comes to celebrity reporting, *Cosmopolitan* tends to present news about celebrities suffering from mental illness more as traditional gossip concerned mostly with what a particular celebrity has been up to, whereas *Teen Vogue* often provides critical context and uses it as a pedagogic tool to talk about everyone who is afflicted by a specific diagnosis. For example, both outlets reported on a series of tweets made by model and actress Cara Delevingne in April 2016 where she wrote about her experience of depression.[95] In the tweets in question, Delevingne clarifies rumors about her quitting modeling, that followed after she had previously spoken out about being depressed while modeling and having shifted to do more acting work. She wrote "I do not blame the fashion industry for anything" and "I suffer from depression and was a model during a particularly rough patch of self hatred." This was followed by two more tweets elaborating on her experience: "I am so lucky for the work I get to do but I used to work to try and escape and just ended up completely exhausting myself" and then "I am focusing on filming and trying to learn how to not pick apart my every flaw. I am really good at that." *Cosmopolitan's* reporting about Delevingne's Twitter activity focuses primarily on what she has to say about the modeling industry.[96] Their article starts with a brief summary of the acting work Delevingne has done recently and the rumors about her quitting modeling. Next it features all of Delevingne's relevant tweets (six in total) embedded into the article, before including a previous quote from the model/actress about suffering from depression. It then concludes by stating that Delevingne is back to modeling again, referencing an announcement that she would be the "new face" of fashion brand Saint Laurent and including two Instagram posts from the model/actress with photos from the campaign.

In contrast, the *Teen Vogue* article about the same tweets starts off by mentioning Delevingne's history of speaking about depression, stating in the first paragraph that "Being skinny and pretty, Cara has said, doesn't mean you can't be depressed, nor does having a successful career you love." After embedding four of the tweets and quoting the one specifically about depression in the text, the *Teen Vogue* writer cites research that "shows that depression is a disorder of the brain," before elaborating:

> Some research suggests that depression is caused by an imbalance of neurotransmitters, the chemicals nerve cells use to talk to each other, while other research puts some of the blame on genetics. This means that depression can affect anyone, no matter how seemingly lucky, successful, or beautiful they are.[97]

The paragraph includes hyperlinks to one article from *Psych Central* and one from *Nature: International weekly journal of science* to back up the claims.[98] What McNamara does here is validate Delevingne's experience by evoking science and biomedicine to explain why someone who seemingly "has it all" can develop depression. It also becomes a pedagogical moment about the causes of the diagnosis.

McNamara then quotes Delevingne when she previously spoke about her depression, before embedding Delevingne's tweet about turning to work as an escape. She then ends the piece with the model/actress' last tweet, which states "I am focusing on filming and trying to learn how to not pick apart my every flaw. I am really good at that" and comments "That's an important lesson to learn. Self-love is a journey, and so is depression. The good news is, neither is a journey you have to take alone."[99] The *Teen Vogue* piece adopts a caring tone that assumes that the reader is not only interested in the fact that a famous model and actress has been depressed, but also in what it means to be depressed and how one might get out of it.

Another instance of celebrity reporting that reveals the different orientations of the magazines is the coverage of artist Mariah Carey's revelation of living with bipolar II disorder in April 2018. The singer opened up in an interview with the celebrity magazine *People* and both *Cosmo* and *Teen Vogue* published their own articles recapping what she had revealed to the other magazine (a common form of celebrity reporting).[100] The two outlets use several of the same quotes from Carey and provide the same general background facts: the singer was first diagnosed in 2001 but did not seek treatment until recently, after having experienced "the hardest couple of years" she had ever been through. *Teen Vogue's* piece, however, is almost twice the length of *Cosmo's* and provides context to both mental health stigma and the bipolar II diagnosis. The *Teen Vogue* article starts with a three-sentence paragraph about the stigma surrounding mental health. Here the author describes how stigma might make the one suffering "feel isolated, ashamed, and even terrified that no one else can understand your internal struggles" and clarifies that mental illnesses "don't discriminate, and truly can affect anyone and everyone, including celebrities who might seem to have 'perfect' lives."[101] Carey and her newly revealed diagnosis are not named until the second paragraph, where the facts of her case are stated. The *Cosmo* article, on the other hand, gets straight to the point as it starts with a two-sentence paragraph that states when Carey first got her diagnosis and that she did not get treatment at the time. In *Cosmo* stigma is only mentioned indirectly when the singer is quoted as having said "I'm hopeful we can get to a place where the stigma is lifted from people going through anything alone," but the magazine does not provide its own commentary on the issue of mental health stigma, like *Teen Vogue* does.

The two publications differ also in how they write about Carey's specific diagnosis. *Teen Vogue* introduces the issue as follows:

> She specifically struggles with bipolar II disorder, which involves periods of depression and hypomania, and is different than bipolar I. According to the National Institute of Mental Health (NIMH), bipolar II is 'defined by a pattern of depressive episodes and hypomanic episodes, but not full-blown manic episodes.'[102]

In this paragraph the phrase "bipolar II disorder" links to the WebMD site for this specific diagnosis and the title "National Institute of Mental Health" links to that organization's information page for the broader spectrum of bipolar disorder. In the *Cosmo* article, the only definition of bipolar II that is given is that it "involves depression and hypomania."[103]

Teen Vogue here seems concerned to give its readers direct information about what bipolar II disorder entails, including differentiating it from other bipolar diagnoses, as well as directing them to sites with more medical facts about the issue, including treatment options. *Cosmo*, on the other hand, is not as concerned about such details, assuming the reader knows or does not care about the difference between bipolar I and II, or what depression and hypomania entail.

This speaks to the difference between the two publications when it comes to providing definitions of the ailments that are discussed. As mentioned above, clinical diagnoses are mentioned in the majority of pieces in both outlets from 2015 and onwards, which seems to suggest that the medical discourses around mental health became more mainstream and were assumed to be widely known from then on. In *Teen Vogue* the mention of clinical diagnoses is repeatedly accompanied by direct definitions of diagnoses, like the ones above, with links to medical sites like WebMD or featuring a quote from an expert (such as a doctor or counselor). This happens in 9% of the *Teen Vogue* articles, which is not an overwhelming amount, but compares to zero such instances in *Cosmopolitan*. In the latter outlet the definitional work is instead happening indirectly in the various ways the issues are being presented. As in the listicles discussed above, for example, the reader gets an idea of what it entails to be depressed or anxious by reading each item on the list. This is also pedagogical in that it provides symptoms and definitions, but these come primarily from the *Cosmo* writers' personal experiences and not from experts or textbook definitions as in *Teen Vogue*.

A CRITICAL AND A NOT-SO-CRITICAL STANCE TOWARD THE PHARMACEUTICAL INDUSTRY

Another example that highlights the differences between the magazines is found in both of their coverage of a research report about the antidepressant drug Paroxetine, which is sold under the brand name Paxil. Comparing how the two outlets choose to write about it shows *Teen Vogue*'s critical stance and *Cosmo*'s lack of one.

The study in question was a reevaluation of a study about the efficacy and harms of Paxil in the treatment of major depression in teens that was conducted in North America from 1994 to 1998 and published as an article in the *Journal of the American Academy of Child and Adolescent Psychiatry* (JAACAP) in 2001.[104] This study, named study 329, was funded by the pharmaceutical company that produced the drug, GlaxoSmithKline (GSK), and concluded that Paxil was safe and efficient for use by children and teenagers (despite the drug only having received FDA-approval for adult use). Study 329 was then used by GSK from 1998-2003 to market the "off-label" use of Paxil in the treatment of children and adolescents, resulting in more than two million prescriptions being made out to teens in 2002 alone.[105] The study became controversial early on, with a FDA officer writing in a formal review of the trial that "on balance, this trial should be considered as a failed trial, in that neither active treatment group showed superiority over placebo by a statistically significant margin."[106] It was then revealed that the paper published in JAACAP under the name of 22 academics, with Brown University's then chief of psychiatry Martin Keller as the lead author, was in fact written by a PR firm hired by GSK and had been composed so as to downplay the negative effects of the drug.[107] In 2004 the FDA even added an explicit warning against prescribing Paxil to children and teens due to the risk of suicidal ideation and self-harm.[108] And in 2012 the US Department of Justice settled a lawsuit against GSK where they pleaded guilty to fraud in their off-label marketing of Paxil and other drugs, paying a record breaking $3 billion in fines.[109]

The study that was being covered by *Cosmopolitan* and *Teen Vogue* was published in 2015 and looks at the raw data behind the original study 329, definitely concluding that Paxil is no more efficient at treating depression in teens and kids than a placebo and that it can potentially lead to suicide and self-harm.[110] What is interesting for the purposes of this discussion is the way the different magazines write about this research. *Cosmopolitan's* piece is titled "This Really Common Antidepressant Could Cause Life-Threatening Side Effects" and starts by stating "Chances are you know someone who takes some sort of medication to treat depression" before briefly accounting for the results of the study. In the fourth paragraph the article addresses the reader directly and states "if you're currently taking Paxil, you probably don't give AF [a fuck] about how or why the original analysis went wrong—you're wondering whether you should trash your prescription."[111] The question is answered firmly in the following paragraph: "The definitive answer is 'no'" followed by an explanation of how sudden withdrawal can increase risk of suicide, and a clarification that Paxil and other SSRIs are not being banned but that more research is called for. And if that was not enough, the piece ends with a clear injunction to only change your medications if there is a problem:

So if you've been taking Paxil for more than a few weeks and you're feeling perfectly fine, there's no reason to freak out—it's unlikely you'll have any problems on your current dose. But if your antidepressant medication is making you feel way worse, talk to the doctor who prescribed it ASAP.[112]

Interestingly, the *Cosmopolitan* writer only mentions that the study had to do with teenage consumers of Paxil briefly when explaining that the new research "re-examined the medical records of 275 adolescent patients with major depression who were involved in the original study." This leaves the impression that the research applies to all takers of the drug, even though the dangers being laid out in the reevaluation of the original Study 329 only applies to teenagers, and not to adult consumers.

The *Teen Vogue* article about the study instead puts the adolescent aspect front and center with the headline "A Popular Antidepressant Is Actually Deadly for Teens." The writer of the piece, Julie Pennell, also highlights the malpractice of the drug company behind Paxil, starting the article with the following statement:

When you aren't feeling well and need to get better, you look to your doctor to make sure you get the right medicine. Your doctor looks at research to make sure he or she gives you the right prescription, but what if the research they're presented with is sneakily flawed?[113]

Pennell then attempts to account for the troubled history of study 329 and the marketing of Paxil to children and teens. She does this by mentioning pharmaceutical company GSK by name, that they were the ones funding the research, and then presented it to downplay the risks and used it to push for the off-label use of the drug. The article also refers to the $3 billion fine paid by the company and the FDA warnings about the potential suicide risk for teens and children taking Paxil. *Cosmopolitan* did not mention any of these specific factors and only vaguely criticized how the pharmaceutical company acted by including a quote from one of the researchers behind the new study saying the findings reveal "how industry hypes drug benefits that might not exist and goes about hiding harms."[114]

In the *Teen Vogue* article Pennell explains that the drug is still available for adults to use and then states:

drug companies are trying to change the law around marketing their medications for off-label uses. Seeing how dangerous Paxil could be for teens however, this can be a very slippery slope. Make sure that you research the medication your doctor prescribes to you, and even get a second opinion.[115]

And after citing the *New York Times* on links between psychiatric drugs and violent acts including suicide (but also mentioning that experts say that there is not enough correlation to draw a straight line between drugs and action), she ends the article stating that "this is scary, and incredibly disheartening to hear that a major drug company would gamble with the lives of teens just for profits." Not only is the tone in this piece serious in *Teen Vogue*'s typical way, but it is also pointedly critical of this particular drug company and the pharmaceutical industry in general.

While the *Cosmopolitan* article focused primarily on the individual aspects of taking the drug, directly encouraging their readers to question Paxil only if they had had problems while taking it, the *Teen Vogue* piece highlights the role of the pharmaceutical company in a much clearer way. Like this, the latter outlet gives the reader a more comprehensive picture of all of the actors involved in developing and prescribing psychiatric medication.

This is also an example of *Teen Vogue* reporting on new research and not taking the findings at hand solely at their face value, but adding critique that puts them in perspective. In a similar vein, the outlet reported on new research that showed depression can cause physical pain in March 2016, and here the author points out that "while people with depression have known for a long time that the disorder affects the whole body, this is the first study to prove that depression is actually a systemic disease rather than just a mental one."[116] Here *Teen Vogue* points to the discrepancies between the firsthand knowledge of many folks living with depression (about the physical effects of depression) and scientific research about the diagnosis. This becomes an indirect critique of the sometimes-narrow frame of health research and foregrounds the lived experience of depression in favor of a blind trust in scientific institutions.

Another example comes from *Teen Vogue*'s reporting on research about depression and suicide rates among transgender kids, rates which the study at hand suggests can be lowered if trans kids are given support and shown acceptance. The *Teen Vogue* writer importantly points out that this disproves "theories that being transgender is inherently bad for mental health" and adds "though many didn't need research to tell them to accept their family members, neighbors, friends, or community members who are transgender, we now have the numbers to tell those who do."[117] Here McNamara manages to bring attention to the connection between mental health and structural discrimination, implicitly showing how transphobia directly affects the psychic wellbeing of transgender persons. In this way *Teen Vogue* might be seen as modeling a way of responsibly reporting on mental illness and its correlation with structural discrimination.

CONCLUSION

In this chapter I have discussed the differences in style, tone, narrative, mode of address, and types of pedagogy and support around depression, anxiety, and general mental health in *Cosmopolitan* and *Teen Vogue*. The general increase in coverage in both outlets and the mention of specific diagnoses from 2015 and onwards suggests that mental illnesses were considered to be obvious aspects of contemporary life from that point on. This is significant because in previous eras mental health and illness have been stigmatized subjects that have not been acknowledged as parts of everyday life, and women's magazines have tended to focus on the positive and upbeat, rather than the negative aspects of life.

In *Cosmopolitan*, the tone tended to be lighthearted, distanced, and relatable, following the magazine's brand of a tongue-in-cheek approach to all aspects of life. Here the relatable self[118] that acknowledges the difficulties of contemporary life in a nonthreatening way is clearly present, especially in the outlet's listicles that frequently use humor to disarm the seriousness of the topics covered. The approach here was often one that presented mental illness as both exceptional and common, clearly marked as different than "just being sad" but also as common as any physical illness. The *Cosmo* pieces that did take a more serious tone were the personal stories that tended to follow the victim-to-victor narrative found in anti-stigma campaigns, where the protagonist starts out by suffering, then receives a diagnosis, and is finally salvaged by the help of medication and therapy. In addition to constructing psychiatry and psychology as the saviors, as traditional anti-stigma narratives, *Cosmo* offered examples that instead constructed mediated technologies like YouTube as the primary mode of support from suffering.

The overall tone in *Teen Vogue* was more serious, shown in the prevalence of general interest stories, a recurring critical perspective, the focus on support, and the direct alignment with mental health awareness and advocacy discourses. By placing general interest stories, such as the one about incarcerated teen Bresha Meadows, alongside more personal and individual-focused pieces the reader learns to include also structural issues in the scope of mental health. The *Teen Vogue* pieces also tend to include critical commentary in addition to the straightforward reporting, which becomes a pedagogical moment about not only the prevalence and causes of various mental illnesses but also their connections to structural issues such as mass incarceration and racial oppression.

A comparison of how the two outlets covered the same celebrity events and science report further showed their differences in tone. Here it became clear that *Teen Vogue* tended to provide readers with more context to the issues affecting the celebrities discussed, whereas *Cosmo* treated them more as traditional celebrity reporting about the specific events that passed. In their coverage of the Paxil study, *Cosmopolitan* wrote about the report in general terms that briefly accounted for the new research findings before advising their readers to only switch medications if they were having issues. *Teen Vogue* on the other hand took a critical stance toward the pharmaceutical company responsible for the deceptive marketing of the drug and accounted for several of the details about the legislative challenges to the company and the study, as well as the general practice of pharmaceutical companies prioritizing profits over individuals' health matters. Like this, the latter outlet gives their readers a comprehensive picture of all of the actors involved in developing and prescribing psychiatric medication and encourages them to adopt a critical and "woke" mindset toward "big pharma."

The examination of these publications' mental health coverage shows that while *Cosmopolitan* tended to follow a script for postfeminist media—full of contradictions, covering serious topics in a tongue-in-cheek way that undermined any gravity, *Teen Vogue* did offer a more nuanced portrayal of mental illness that incited its readers to a more critical and engaged interpretation of dominant mental health paradigms. In this sense *Cosmo* provides an example of profitable vulnerability in that it aligns itself with the trendy themes of depression, anxiety, and other diagnoses, while maintaining a comfortable distance that avoids striking a too somber or heavy tone. The vulnerability acknowledged here is one that largely has already been dealt with or is one step on the road toward becoming confident and resilient again.[119] *Teen Vogue*, on the other hand, does offer more spacious definitions of mental illness that does not shy away from difficult conversations. With their focus on support and their providing of resources (such as hotline numbers), they instead can be seen as giving their readers life-saving information to assist in bettering their mental health. They are then more aligned with the critical sad girl culture found on social media and discussed in Chap. 5.

The study of *Cosmopolitan's* and *Teen Vogue's* approach to mental health during this time further underscores the increase in conversations around mental health from 2015 and onwards. As I will discuss further in the following chapter in relation to celebrities, this can be tied to changes in branding strategies when it comes to relatability. In a changing media landscape, where social media is dominating more and more of people's media consumption, traditional media outlets like the ones discussed here also turn to more intimate themes and topics, of which mental illness is the latest addition.

NOTES

1. Duffy, *Remake, Remodel*, 3.
2. McRobbie, "Jackie Magazine."
3. Ibid, 69.
4. Duffy, *Remake, Remodel*.
5. Ballaster et al., *Women's Worlds*; Currie, *Girl Talk*; Ferguson, *Forever Feminine*; Gough-Yates, *Understanding Women's Magazines*; McCracken, *Decoding Women's Magazines*.
6. Bordo, *Unbearable Weight*; Wolf, *The Beauty Myth*.
7. Bhattacharyya, *Sexuality and Society*; Jeffreys, *Beauty and Misogyny*; Onwurah, "Sexist, Racist and Above All Capitalist."
8. McRobbie, *The Aftermath of Feminism*.
9. Gill, "Post-Postfeminism?;" Orgad and Gill, *Confidence Culture*.
10. Gill, "Mediated Intimacy and Postfeminism," 365.
11. Ibid.
12. Ibid, 362.
13. Ibid, 362.
14. Coulter and Moruzi, "Woke Girls," 6.
15. My analysis involved categorizing the articles in each outlet according to the form they took, and I refer to percentages throughout this chapter which largely refers back to this analytical work.
16. Hill, "Ask Logan;" Simmons, "Ask Rachel."
17. Barker, Gill, and Harvey, *Mediated Intimacy*; Ouellette and Hay, *Better Living Through Reality TV*.
18. Zimmerman, "How Cosmo Conquered the World."
19. Machin and Thornborrow, "Branding and Discourse: The Case of Cosmopolitan."
20. Ibid, 454.
21. Poole, "Top nine things you need to know about 'listicles.'"
22. Breslaw, "10 Things You Should Never Say To Someone With Depression;" Koman, "10 Things You Should Never Say To Someone With Anxiety."
23. Dingle, "17 Things to Never Say to a Girl With Borderline Personality Disorder;" Koman, "13 Things Not to Say to Someone Who Is Stressed Out;" Peyser, "10 Things You Should Not Say To Someone With An Eating Disorder."

24. Breslaw, "10 Things You Should Never Say To Someone With Depression," italicization in original.
25. Peyser, "16 Things Only Girls On Antidepressants Will Understand;" Peyser, "14 Struggles Only Girls With Anxiety Will Understand;" Peyser, "12 Struggles Only Girls With Depression Will Understand."
26. Smothers, "17 Dating Struggles Girls With Anxiety Understand;" Pugachevsky, "12 Dating Struggles Only Girls With ADHD Will Understand."
27. Peyser, "16 Things Only Girls On Antidepressants Will Understand," italicization in original.
28. Machin and Thornborrow, "Branding and Discourse: The Case of Cosmopolitan." I return to the function of humor in relation to mental health in Chap. 5, where I discuss how humor is used among social media users writing about their sadness and various mental illnesses diagnoses online.
29. Moore, "13 Things I Wish I Knew About Depression When I Was a Teenager."
30. Peyser, "12 Struggles Only Girls With Depression Will Understand."
31. Breslaw, "10 Things You Should Never Say To Someone With Depression."
32. Moore, "13 Things I Wish I Knew About Depression When I Was a Teenager."
33. Breslaw, "10 Things You Should Never Say To Someone With Depression."
34. Blackman, "Psychiatric culture and bodies of resistance."
35. Kanai, "Girlfriendship and sameness;" Kanai, "The best friend, the boyfriend, other girls, hot guys, and creeps;" Kanai, *Gender and Relatability in Digital Culture.*
36. Gill and Kanai, "Mediating Neoliberal Capitalism," 321.
37. Ibid, 322.
38. Peyser, "16 Things Only Girls On Antidepressants Will Understand," italicization in original.
39. Blackman, "Psychiatric culture and bodies of resistance."
40. Justich, "Why I Turn to YouTube When My Anxiety Gets Out of Control."
41. Ibid.
42. Blackman, "Self-help, media cultures and the production of female psychopathology;" Hochschild, "The Commercial Spirit of Intimate Life."
43. Hochschild, "The Commercial Spirit of Intimate Life," 3.
44. Ibid, 13, italicization in original.
45. Ibid, 13.
46. Ibid, 14.

47. Blackman, "Self-help, media cultures and the production of female psychopathology," 225.
48. Ibid, 225.
49. SACCONEJOLYs, Youtube channel, accessed June 27, 2022, https://www.youtube.com/c/sacconejolys.
50. Justich, "Why I Turn to YouTube When My Anxiety Gets Out of Control."
51. Banet-Weiser, *Empowered*.
52. Blackman, "Self-help, media cultures and the production of female psychopathology," 230.
53. Epstein, "How to Beat the Winter Blues."
54. That year 35% of their articles mention a clinical diagnosis, which goes up to 61% in 2014, 78% in 2015 and 2016, down to 77% in 2017, and then up to 81% in 2018.
55. Koman, "This Mom's Powerful Selfie Proves There's No Shame in Taking Anxiety Medication."
56. Coulter and Moruzi, "Woke Girls," 6.
57. Banet-Weiser, *Empowered*, 103.
58. Duca, "Donald Trump Is Gaslighting America."
59. Banet-Weiser, *Empowered*, 104.
60. Teen Vogue, website, accessed June 27, 2022, https://www.teen-vogue.com.
61. Hinchliffe, "The dissonance between Vogue and Teen Vogue is finally too loud to ignore."
62. Coulter and Moruzi, "Woke Girls," 1.
63. Ibid, 7.
64. Pulliam-Moore, "How 'woke' went from black activist watchword to teen internet slang."
65. Ashlee, Zamora, and Karikari, "We are woke," 90.
66. Coulter and Moruzi, "Woke Girls," 7.
67. Ibid, 7.
68. McNamara, "Accepting Transgender Kids Will Lower Depression and Suicide Rates;" McNamara, "Majority of Americans Say Racial Discrimination Is the Cause of Their Rising Stress."
69. Sinay, "'Telepsychiatry' Lets Therapists Treat Your Mental Health Over Skype, FaceTime;" McNamara, "Hospital Gets Sued for Discrimination After Transgender Teen Suicide."
70. McNamara, "Bresha Meadows Will Be Transferred to a Mental Health Facility."
71. Justice Policy Institute, "Incarcerating Youth can Aggravate Crime and Frustrate Education, Employment and Health for Young People."
72. McNamara, "Bresha Meadows Will Be Transferred to a Mental Health Facility."

73. Quinn, "26 Date Ideas for Your Anxious Partner."
74. 6% of the *Teen Vogue* articles are collaborations with this site.
75. Blades, "11 Things You Can Do To Help Black Lives Matter End Police Violence."
76. Szpitalak, "11 Things You Can Do to Avoid Self-Harm."
77. Ibid.
78. Ibid.
79. Mei, "Demi Lovato Opens Up About Her Struggles with Addiction, Bulimia, and Bipolar Disorder;" Narins "This Really Common Antidepressant Could Cause Life-Threatening Side Effects;" Peyser, "What I Learned From Posting About My Mental Illness on Social Media."
80. In 2015 70% of their articles mention a clinical diagnosis, which goes up to 82% in 2016, 93% in 2017, and down to 91% in 2018.
81. This kind of explicit definitions appear in 9% of their pieces.
82. Ceron, "This Might Be Why Liam Payne Cancelled One Direction's Concert On Tuesday."
83. ADAA, "Anxiety Disorders - Facts & Statistics," website, accessed June 25, 2022, https://adaa.org/understanding-anxiety/facts-statistics.
84. Saint Louis, "For Families of Teens at Suicide Risk."
85. Cline, "This Is What's Missing From '13 Reasons Why,'" italicization in original.
86. Ibid.
87. Gross, "What Teens Think of '13 Reasons Why.'"
88. McNamara, "Mental Health Resources For People Triggered By '13 Reasons Why.'"
89. Brito, "Netflix deletes Hannah Baker death scene in Season 1 finale;" Herman, "Survivors Explain What Was Wrong With the '13 Reasons Why' Suicide Scene."
90. Spector, "Why mental health advocates use the words 'died by suicide.'"
91. McNamara, "Lady Gaga Penned a Letter About Living With PTSD."
92. *Teen Vogue*, "Days Derailed: The Coronavirus Crisis," website, accessed June 28, 2022, https://www.teenvogue.com/collection/coronavirus.
93. Aronowitz, "Dating and Coronavirus;" Diavolo, "Coronavirus and COVID-19;" Flynn, "What to Do if You're Isolated With an Abuser During the Coronavirus Crisis;" McNamara, "Coronavirus Anxiety."
94. Mallett, "The Coronavirus Pandemic Demonstrates the Failures of Capitalism;" Nasheed, "The Coronavirus Is Killing Black Americans In Alarming Numbers."
95. McNamara, "Cara Delevingne Takes to Twitter to Talk About Her Depression;" Storey, "Cara Delevingne Opens Up About Depression."
96. Storey, "Cara Delevingne Opens Up About Depression."
97. McNamara, "Cara Delevingne Takes to Twitter to Talk About Her Depression."

98. Hyman, "Mental health: Depression needs large human-genetics studies;" Spielmans, "Research Updates: Depression."

99. McNamara, "Cara Delevingne Takes to Twitter to Talk About Her Depression."

100. Baty, "Mariah Carey Opens up About Her Struggle With Bipolar Disorder;" Belle, "Mariah Carey Opened Up About Having Bipolar Disorder."

101. Belle, "Mariah Carey Opened Up About Having Bipolar Disorder."

102. Ibid.

103. Baty, "Mariah Carey Opens up About Her Struggle With Bipolar Disorder."

104. Keller et al, "Efficacy of Paroxetine in the Treatment of Adolescent Major Depression;" Le Noury et al, "Restoring Study 329."

105. Doshi, "No correction, no retraction, no apology, no comment."

106. Mosholder, "Clinical Review: Paxil."

107. Doshi, "No correction, no retraction, no apology, no comment."

108. Belluz, "Researchers said a popular antidepressant was safe for teens."

109. U.S. Department of Justice, "GlaxoSmithKline to Plead Guilty and Pay $3 Billion to Resolve Fraud Allegations and Failure to Report Safety Data."

110. Le Noury et al, "Restoring Study 329."

111. Narins, "This Really Common Antidepressant Could Cause Life-Threatening Side Effects."

112. Ibid.

113. Pennell, "A Popular Antidepressant Is Actually Deadly for Teens."

114. Narins, "This Really Common Antidepressant Could Cause Life-Threatening Side Effects."

115. Pennell, "A Popular Antidepressant Is Actually Deadly for Teens."

116. McNamara, "Depression Causes Physical Pain."

117. McNamara, "Accepting Transgender Kids Will Lower Depression and Suicide Rates."

118. Kanai, *Gender and Relatability in Digital Culture*; Gill and Kanai, "Mediating Neoliberal Capitalism."

119. Orgad and Gill, *Confidence Culture*; McRobbie, *Feminism and the Politics of Resilience*.

References

Aronowitz, Nona Willis. "Dating and Coronavirus: Can You Still Kiss, Have Sex, and Go on Dates During Social Distancing?" *Teen Vogue*, March 18, 2020. https://www.teenvogue.com/story/dating-and-coronavirus.

Ashlee, Aeriel A., Bianca Zamora, and Shamika N. Karikari. "We Are Woke: A Collaborative Critical Autoethnography of Three 'Womxn' of Color Graduate Students in Higher Education." *International Journal of Multicultural Education* 19, no. 1 (2017): 89–104. https://doi.org/10.18251/ijme.v19i1.1259.

Ballaster, Ros, Margaret Beetham, Elizabeth Frazer, and Sandra Hebron. *Women's Worlds: Ideology, Femininity, and the Woman's Magazine*. London: Macmillan, 1991.

Banet-Weiser, Sarah. *Empowered: Popular Feminism and Popular Misogyny*. Durham and London: Duke University Press, 2018.

Barker, Meg-John, Rosalind Gill, and Laura Harvey. *Mediated Intimacy: Sex Advice in Media Culture*. Cambridge: Polity, 2018.

Baty, Emma. "Mariah Carey Opens up About Her Struggle with Bipolar Disorder." *Cosmopolitan*, April 11, 2018. https://www.cosmopolitan.com/entertainment/celebs/a19743108/mariah-carey-bipolar-disorder/

Belle, Elly. "Mariah Carey Opened Up About Having Bipolar Disorder." *Teen Vogue*, April 11, 2018. https://www.teenvogue.com/story/mariah-carey-bipolar-disorder.

Belluz, Julia. "Researchers Said a Popular Antidepressant Was Safe for Teens. It Was Actually Deadly." *Vox*, September 19, 2015. https://www.vox.com/2015/9/19/9355121/paxil-research-fraud.

Bhattacharyya, Gargi. *Sexuality and Society: An Introduction*. London: Routledge, 2002.

Blackman, Lisa. "Psychiatric Culture and Bodies of Resistance." *Body & Society* 13, no. 2 (2007): 1–23. https://doi.org/10.1177/1357034X07077770.

Blackman, Lisa. "Self-Help, Media Cultures and the Production of Female Psychopathology." *Cultural Studies* 7, no. 2 (2004): 219–36.

Blades, Lincoln Anthony. "10 Things You Can Do to Help Black Lives Matter End Police Violence." *Teen Vogue*, July 9, 2016. https://www.teenvogue.com/story/support-the-black-lives-matter-movement.

Bordo, Susan. *Unbearable Weight: Feminism, Western Culture, and the Body*. Tenth anni. Berkeley, Los Angeles, London: University of California Press, 2003.

Breslaw, Anna. "10 Things You Should Never Say To Someone With Depression." *Cosmopolitan*, December 19, 2013. https://www.cosmopolitan.com/sex-love/advice/a5215/things-not-to-say-depression/.

Brito, Christopher. "Netflix Deletes Hannah Baker Death Scene in Season 1 Finale." *CBSNews.Com*, July 16, 2019. https://www.cbsnews.com/news/13-reasons-why-suicide-scene-hannah-baker-season-finale-death-katherine-langford-season-1-episode-13/.

Ceron, Ella. "This Might Be Why Liam Payne Cancelled One Direction's Concert on Tuesday." *Teen Vogue*, October 22, 2015. https://www.teenvogue.com/story/liam-payne-anxiety-attack.

Cline, MollyKate. "This Is What's Missing From '13 Reasons Why.'" *Teen Vogue*, March 31, 2017. https://www.teenvogue.com/story/what-netflix-thirteen-reasons-missing-mental-health.

Coulter, Natalie, and Kristine Moruzi. "Woke Girls: From The Girl's Realm to Teen Vogue." *Feminist Media Studies* 00, no. 00 (2020): 1–15. https://doi.org/https://doi.org/10.1080/14680777.2020.1736119.

Currie, Dawn. *Girl Talk: Adolescent Magazines and Their Readers.* Toronto: University of Toronto Press, 1999.

Diavolo, Lucy. "Coronavirus and COVID-19: What They Are, What's the Difference, and How You Can Respond." *Teen Vogue*, March 12, 2020. https://www.teenvogue.com/story/coronavirus-covid-19-101-explainer.

Dingle, Charlotte. "17 Things to Never Say to a Girl with Borderline Personality Disorder." *Cosmopolitan*, March 6, 2016. https://www.cosmopolitan.com/health-fitness/a54813/things-to-never-say-borderline-personality-disorder/.

Doshi, Peter. "No Correction, No Retraction, No Apology, No Comment: Paroxetine Trial Reanalysis Raises Questions about Institutional Responsibility." *BMJ (Clinical Research Ed.)* 351 (September 16, 2015): h4629. https://doi.org/10.1136/bmj.h4629.

Duca, Lauren. "Donald Trump Is Gaslighting America." *Teen Vogue*, December 10, 2016. https://www.teenvogue.com/story/donald-trump-is-gaslighting-america.

Duffy, Brooke Erin. *Remake, Remodel: Women's Magazines in the Digital Age.* Urbana, Chicago and Springfield: University of Illinois Press, 2013.

Epstein, Leonora. "How to Beat the Winter Blues." *Cosmopolitan*, January 30, 2009. https://www.cosmopolitan.com/lifestyle/advice/a2815/beat-the-winter-blues/.

Ferguson, Marjorie. *Forever Feminine: Women's Magazines and the Cult of Femininity.* London: Heinemann, 1983.

Flynn, Caitlin. "What to Do If You're Isolated With an Abuser During the Coronavirus Crisis." *Teen Vogue*, April 2, 2020. https://www.teenvogue.com/story/what-to-do-if-youre-isolated-with-an-abuser-during-the-coronavirus-crisis.

Gill, Rosalind. "Post-Postfeminism?: New Feminist Visibilities in Postfeminist Times." *Feminist Media Studies* 16, no. 4 (2016): 610–30. https://doi.org/10.1080/14680777.2016.1193293.

Gill, Rosalind. "Mediated Intimacy and Postfeminism: A Discourse Analytic Examination of Sex and Relationships Advice in a Women's Magazine." *Discourse & Communication* 3, no. 4 (2009): 345–69. https://doi.org/10.1177/1750481309343870.

Gill, Rosalind, and Akane Kanai. "Mediating Neoliberal Capitalism: Affect, Subjectivity and Inequality." *Journal of Communication* 68, no. 2 (2018): 318–26. https://doi.org/10.1093/joc/jqy002.

Gough-Yates, Anna. *Understanding Women's Magazines: Publishing, Markets and Readerships.* London: Routledge, 2003.

Gross, Elana. "What Teens Think of '13 Reasons Why.'" *Teen Vogue*, May 17, 2017. https://www.teenvogue.com/story/what-teens-think-thirteen-reasons-why.

Herman, Lily. "Survivors Explain What Was Wrong With the '13 Reasons Why' Suicide Scene." *Teen Vogue*, June 15, 2017. https://www.teenvogue.com/story/survivors-explain-what-was-wrong-with-13-reasons-why-suicide-scene.

Hill, Logan. "Ask Logan: My Boyfriend Is Super Rude to Me Whenever He Plays Video Games." *Cosmopolitan*, May 17, 2017. https://www.cosmopolitan.com/sex-love/a9660873/ask-logan-video-games-long-distance-mental-health/.

Hochschild, Arlie Russell. "The Commercial Spirit of Intimate Life." *Theory, Culture & Society* 11 (1994): 1–24.

Hyman, Steven. "Mental Health: Depression Needs Large Human-Genetics Studies." *Nature: International Weekly Journal of Science*. Nature Publishing Group, November 13, 2014. https://doi.org/10.1038/515189a.

Jeffreys, Sheila. *Beauty and Misogyny: Harmful Cultural Practices in the West.* London: Routledge, 2005.

Justice Policy Institute. "Incarcerating Youth Can Aggravate Crime and Frustrate Education, Employment and Health for Young People." *Justice Policy Institute*, November 28, 2006. http://www.justicepolicy.org/news/1977.

Kanai, Akane. "The Best Friend, the Boyfriend, Other Girls, Hot Guys, and Creeps: The Relational Production of Self on Tumblr." *Feminist Media Studies* 17, no. 6 (2017a): 911–25. https://doi.org/10.1080/14680777.2017.1298647.

Kanai, Akane. "Girlfriendship and Sameness: Affective Belonging in a Digital Intimate Public." *Journal of Gender Studies* 26, no. 3 (2017b): 293–306. https://doi.org/10.1080/09589236.2017.1281108.

Kanai, Akane. *Gender and Relatability in Digital Culture: Managing Affect, Intimacy and Value.* Cham: Palgrave Macmillan, 2019.

Keller, Martin B., Neal D. Ryan, Michael Strober, Rachel G. Klein, Stan P. Kutcher, Boris Birmaher, Owen R. Hagino, et al. "Efficacy of Paroxetine in the Treatment of Adolescent Major Depression: A Randomized, Controlled Trial." *Journal of the American Academy of Child & Adolescent Psychiatry* 40, no. 7 (2001): 762–72. 10.1097/00004583-200107000-00010.

Koman, Tess. "10 Things You Should Never Say To Someone With Anxiety." *Cosmopolitan*, April 23, 2014. https://www.cosmopolitan.com/health-fitness/advice/a6483/things-not-to-say-to-someone-with-anxiety/.

Koman, Tess. "13 Things Not to Say to Someone Who Is Stressed Out." *Cosmopolitan*, June 24, 2015a. https://www.cosmopolitan.com/sex-love/news/a42459/things-not-to-say-to-someone-who-is-stressed-out/.

Koman, Tess. "This Mom's Powerful Selfie Proves There's No Shame in Taking Anxiety Medication." *Cosmopolitan*, September 30, 2015b. https://www.cosmopolitan.com/lifestyle/news/a46992/erin-jones-mighty-and-medicated-selfie/.

Noury, Joanna Le, John M Nardo, David Healy, Jon Jureidini, Melissa Raven, Catalin Tufanaru, and Elia Abi-Jaoude. "Restoring Study 329: Efficacy and Harms of Paroxetine and Imipramine in Treatment of Major Depression in Adolescence." *BMJ* 351 (September 16, 2015): h4320. https://doi.org/10.1136/bmj.h4320.

Machin, David, and Joanna Thornborrow. "Branding and Discourse: The Case of Cosmopolitan." *Discourse and Society* 14, no. 4 (2003): 453–71. https://doi.org/10.1177/0957926503014004003.

Mallett, Kandist. "The Coronavirus Pandemic Demonstrates the Failures of Capitalism." *Teen Vogue*, March 24, 2020. https://www.teenvogue.com/story/coronavirus-pandemic-failures-capitalism.

McCracken, Ellen. *Decoding Women's Magazines: From Mademoiselle to Ms.* Basingstoke: Macmillan, 1993.

McNamara, Brittney. "Accepting Transgender Kids Will Lower Depression and Suicide Rates." *Teen Vogue*, March 1, 2016a. https://www.teenvogue.com/story/transgender-depression-suicide.

McNamara, Brittney. "Majority of Americans Say Racial Discrimination Is the Cause of Their Rising Stress." *Teen Vogue*, March 14, 2016b. https://www.teenvogue.com/story/discrimination-anxiety.

McNamara, Brittney. "Depression Causes Physical Pain." *Teen Vogue*, March 15, 2016c. https://www.teenvogue.com/story/physical-pain-depression-study.

McNamara, Brittney. "Cara Delevingne Takes to Twitter to Talk About Her Depression." *Teen Vogue*, April 1, 2016d. https://www.teenvogue.com/story/cara-delevingne-tweets-depression-modeling.

McNamara, Brittney. "Hospital Gets Sued for Discrimination After Transgender Teen Suicide." *Teen Vogue*, October 3, 2016e. https://www.teenvogue.com/story/transgender-teen-suicide-hospital-sued-after-misgendering.

McNamara, Brittney. "Lady Gaga Penned a Letter About Living With PTSD." *Teen Vogue*, December 7, 2016f. https://www.teenvogue.com/story/lady-gaga-penned-a-letter-about-living-with-ptsd.

McNamara, Brittney. "Bresha Meadows Will Be Transferred to a Mental Health Facility." *Teen Vogue*, January 20, 2017a. https://www.teenvogue.com/story/bresha-meadows-transferred-mental-health-facility.

McNamara, Brittney. "Mental Health Resources for People Triggered By '13 Reasons Why.'" *Teen Vogue*, June 8, 2017b. https://www.teenvogue.com/story/mental-health-resources-for-people-triggered-by-thirteen-reasons-why.

McNamara, Brittney. "Coronavirus Anxiety: How to Cope." *Teen Vogue*, March 10, 2020. https://www.teenvogue.com/story/coronavirus-anxiety.

McRobbie, Angela. "Jackie Magazine: Romantic Individualism and the Teenage Girl." In *Feminism and Youth Culture*, 2nd ed. New York: Routledge, 2000.

McRobbie, Angela. *The Aftermath of Feminism: Gender, Culture and Social Change*. London, Thousand Oaks, New Delhi and Singapore: SAGE, 2009.

Mosholder, Andrew D. "Clinical Review: Paxil," 2002.

Narins, Elizabeth. "This Really Common Antidepressant Could Cause Life-Threatening Side Effects." *Cosmopolitan*, September 17, 2015. https://www.cosmopolitan.com/health-fitness/news/a46421/new-study-finds-a-common-antidepressant-has-a-life-threatening-side-effect/.

Nasheed, Jameelah. "The Coronavirus Is Killing Black Americans In Alarming Numbers." *Teen Vogue*, April 7, 2020. https://www.teenvogue.com/story/black-americans-coronavirus-cases-deaths.

Onwurah, C. "Sexist, Racist and Above All Capitalist: How Women's Magazines Create Media Apartheid." In *Out of Focus: Writings on Women and the Media*, edited by Kath Davies, Julienne Dickey, and Teresa Stratford, 47–52. London: Women's Press, 1987.

Orgad, Shani, and Rosalind Gill. *Confidence Culture*. Durham and London: Duke University Press, 2022. https://doi.org/https://doi.org/10.1215/9781478021834.

Ouellette, Laurie, and James Hay. *Better Living Through Reality TV: Television and Post-Welfare Citizenship*. Malden, MA, Oxford, and Victoria: Blackwell Publishing, 2008.

Pennell, Julie. "A Popular Antidepressant Is Actually Deadly for Teens." *Teen Vogue*, September 21, 2015. https://www.teenvogue.com/story/paxil-unsafe-teenagers-new-research-antidepressants.

Peyser, Eve. "16 Things Only Girls On Antidepressants Will Understand." *Cosmopolitan*, May 6, 2016a. https://www.cosmopolitan.com/sex-love/a58060/the-struggles-of-being-on-antidepressants/.

Peyser, Eve. "14 Things Only Girls With Anxiety Will Understand." *Cosmopolitan*, May 16, 2016b. https://www.cosmopolitan.com/sex-love/news/a58188/struggles-of-having-anxiety/.

Peyser, Eve. "12 Struggles Only Girls With Depression Will Understand." *Cosmopolitan*, May 20, 2016c. https://www.cosmopolitan.com/sex-love/a58752/struggles-of-having-depression/.

Peyser, Eve. "10 Things You Should Not Say To Someone With An Eating Disorder." *Cosmopolitan*, June 3, 2016d. https://www.cosmopolitan.com/sex-love/a59339/things-never-to-say-to-someone-with-an-eating-disorder/.

Poole, Steven. "Top Nine Things You Need to Know about 'Listicles.'" *The Guardian*, November 12, 2013. https://www.theguardian.com/books/2013/nov/12/listicles-articles-written-lists-steven-poole.

Pugachevsky, Julia. "12 Dating Struggles Only Girls With ADHD Understand." *Cosmopolitan*, February 9, 2017. https://www.cosmopolitan.com/sex-love/a8686980/dating-struggles-of-adhd/.

Pulliam-Moore, Charles. "How 'woke' Went from Black Activist Watchword to Teen Internet Slang." *Splinter*, January 8, 2016. https://splinternews.com/how-woke-went-from-black-activist-watchword-to-teen-int-1793853989.

Quinn, Haley. "26 Date Ideas for You or Your Partner With Anxiety." *Teen Vogue*, February 10, 2018. https://www.teenvogue.com/story/26-date-ideas-for-your-anxious-partner.

Saint Louis, Catherine. "For Families of Teens at Suicide Risk, '13 Reasons' Raises Concerns." *New York Times*, May 1, 2017. https://www.nytimes.com/2017/05/01/well/family/for-families-of-teens-at-suicide-risk-13-reasons-triggers-concerns.html.

Simmons, Rachel. "Ask Rachel: I Think My Friend Could Be an Alcoholic." *Teen Vogue*, November 6, 2012. https://www.teenvogue.com/story/friend-becoming-alcoholic.

Sinay, Danielle. "'Telepsychiatry' Lets Therapists Treat Your Mental Health Over Skype, FaceTime." *Teen Vogue*, August 5, 2016. https://www.teenvogue.com/story/telehealth-telepsychiatry-therapy-skype-mental-health.

Smothers, Hannah. "17 Dating Struggles Girls With Anxiety Understand." *Cosmopolitan*, June 6, 2016. https://www.cosmopolitan.com/sex-love/news/a59468/dating-struggles-girls-with-anxiety-understand/.

Spector, Nicole. "Why Mental Health Advocates Use the Words 'Died by Suicide.'" *Nbcnews.Com*, June 6, 2018. https://www.nbcnews.com/better/health/why-mental-health-advocates-use-words-died-suicide-ncna880546.

Spielmans, Glen. "Research Updates: Depression." *Psych Central*, 2015. https://pro.psychcentral.com/research-updates-depression/.

Storey, Kate. "Cara Delevingne Opens Up About Depression." *Cosmopolitan*, April 1, 2016. https://www.cosmopolitan.com/entertainment/news/a56102/cara-delevingne-depression-modeling-tweets/.

Szpitalak, Vijayta. "11 Things You Can Do to Avoid Self-Harm." *Teen Vogue*, May 9, 2016. https://www.teenvogue.com/story/self-harm-alternatives.

U.S. Department of Justice. "GlaxoSmithKline to Plead Guilty and Pay $3 Billion to Resolve Fraud Allegations and Failure to Report Safety Data | OPA | Department of Justice." *U.S. Department of Justice*, July 2, 2012. https://www.justice.gov/opa/pr/glaxosmithkline-plead-guilty-and-pay-3-billion-resolve-fraud-allegations-and-failure-report.

Wolf, Naomi. *The Beauty Myth: How Images of Beauty are Used against Women.* New York: Perennial, 2002.

Zimmerman, Edith. "How Cosmo Conquered the World." *The New York Times*, August 3, 2012. https://www.nytimes.com/2012/08/05/magazine/how-cosmo-conquered-the-world.html.

CHAPTER 4

Celebrity Mental Health: Intimacy, Ordinariness, and Repeated Self-Transformation

While magazines directly (and indirectly) tell us what to do, celebrity reporting functions in a similar pedagogical way by showing audiences how famous people act in certain situations. When celebrities share their personal health struggles, scholars have argued that they serve three main functions: education, inspiration, and activism/advocacy.[1] This is the logic presented at face value by celebrities themselves and those actively telling their stories——that when a famous person comes out and reveals that they are suffering, they communicate to fans that it is okay to feel that way and ideally inspire them to seek help. *Teen Vogue's* insistence on the importance of speaking out and fighting the stigma discussed in the previous chapter is an example of this. So is Lady Gaga's statement in conjunction with revealing that she lives with PTSD that "the most inexpensive and perhaps the best medicine in the world is words."[2] Other scholars have added that celebrity health narratives also do ideological work in that they present "images and ideas about how we should interpret, manage and value mental illness as well as the identities of those who suffer from it."[3]

This chapter focuses on female celebrities[4] who have spoken out about their own mental illness, by looking at the very public struggles of singers Demi Lovato and Selena Gomez. It also briefly discusses the employment of a sad aesthetic by artist Lana del Rey. These cases and the overall rise in celebrity expressions about mental health can be tied to a turn in celebrity branding around authenticity and intimacy. Together with the previous chapter, it shows how media and pop cultural attention to mental health is linked to changes in branding strategies around relatability. This chapter

F. Thelandersson, *21st Century Media and Female Mental Health*,
https://doi.org/10.1007/978-3-031-16756-0_4

shows that, just as there was an increase in magazine coverage of mental illness from 2015 and on, there was a spike in celebrity confessions about various psychiatric diagnoses around this time.

Within the original time frames of this research project, 2008-2018, 105 female celebrities who had spoken out about various experiences of mental illness were identified.[5] Since the original cut-off point, the list has steadily become longer, with more and more famous individuals sharing their struggles with the world. Among these are people like entertainer Paris Hilton (who revealed a traumatic history of childhood abuse), royal Meghan Markle (who in an infamous Oprah interview shared that she had been suicidal), and athlete Naomi Osaka (who took a break from tennis due to mental health issues).[6]

Just as with this book's general scope, the focus here is on American celebrities or those with a global appeal. In the original group of celebrities, 78% were white, 12% black, 5% latinx, and 5% mixed race. In other words, the majority of women celebrities who have spoken out about their mental health are white. The subject that gets to be open about her difficulties, tends to be white or white-passing.

Among the original 105 celebrities, the most common diagnosis mentioned was anxiety, closely followed by depression, as well as those having suffered both anxiety and depression. There were also several accounts of living with postpartum depression and bipolar disorder.[7] Other diagnoses and experiences that occurred were social anxiety, suicidal ideation, self-harm, eating disorders, and obsessive-compulsive disorder (OCD). Among these categories several overlapped, meaning the same person might have talked about having multiple diagnoses. There were also a few cases where stars had only talked about mental health in general, but still made it to several compilation lists of celebrities speaking out, and they are thus also included here.

CHANGES OVER TIME: FROM SPECULATIONS TO CONFESSIONS

The majority of these celebrity confessions took place toward the end of the decade, with a clear increase in 2015 and onwards. The stars included here have all spoken firsthand about their own experiences of depression, anxiety, or other diagnoses. These confessions primarily took place in interviews with magazines, but also at times on social media, with stars revealing diagnoses directly to their fans on their personal accounts, like the case of Cara Delevingne discussed in the previous chapter. Some also happened in memoirs (that were subsequently reported on by media covering celebrities), first-person essays in the popular press, press statements in relation to a rehab or hospital stay, participation in mental health awareness campaigns, on personal apps, and on reality television shows.[8]

Looking at celebrity reporting around 2008–2009, a lot of it was dedicated to female stars who seemed to go through mental distress, but they rarely came forward themselves to speak about what they were dealing with; instead, it was the media speculating about what particular diagnosis someone might have had. This creates a different kind of celebrity health narrative than when the star herself speaks out, since speculations from others always can be denied, but firsthand statements tend to be carefully crafted to fit within the celebrity's overall brand. Su Holmes and Diane Negra have pointed to the "intensely and negatively scrutinizing public gaze [that] was trained so often on female celebrities in a practice that reached fever pitch in 2008."[9] A fever pitch that was not an "accident of historical timing" but a way of misdirecting anxieties and blame for the global financial crisis and instead position "female celebrity as itself an overvalued and depreciating asset."[10] In this way, famous women took the heat for the public's anxieties about the financial system and the tabloidized press used its investigative functions to examine female "trainwrecks" rather than economic institutions.

The trainwrecks that received scrutinized attention were often suspected of suffering from mental health challenges. For example, one of the most closely watched public breakdowns at the start of 2008 was that of singer Britney Spears, which (could be said) to have peaked in February 2007 when she shaved her head in front of scores of paparazzi photographers who spread the news worldwide overnight.[11] During 2008 Spears was committed to a psychiatric ward twice and then put under a conservatorship in which her father Jamie Spears had ultimate authority over her finances and most personal decisions, something she lived with for over 13 years.[12]

2010-2011 saw the peak of former child actor Lindsay Lohan's life descending into chaos, with her spending time in rehab and jail multiple times.[13] Around this time the world also saw singer Amy Winehouse rise to stardom and break down in public, ending with her death by alcohol poisoning in 2011.[14] In 2013 and 2014 former child actor Amanda Bynes went through a very public breakdown involving several highly publicized drug binges and court battles with her parents.[15] Several of these female celebrities appeared among the sad girls on Tumblr that I discuss in the following chapter. On this digital platform users would post images of these stars (often in states of distress) in ways that idolized them and reinforced a melancholic notion of sadness as romantic, mystical, and inspirational.[16]

In most of these cases of public breakdown, the speculations about the famous women's mental health were done by observers and not by the women themselves. What started to change around 2015 was that celebrities themselves began to "come out" and address their own mental health in large numbers. One example of how attitudes about celebrities and mental illness changed toward the end of the decade is singer Mariah Carey's revelation of a bipolar II diagnosis to *People* magazine in April 2018 (the coverage of which I discussed in the previous chapter).[17] Throughout her 25-year career, the singer had gone through two highly publicized marriages, a divorce, and a televised mental breakdown but did not speak out directly about her mental health until 2018, despite having received her diagnosis already in 2001.[18] The case of actress Brittany Snow is another example. She opened up about her experiences of anorexia and depression to *People* magazine in 2007, but the public's reaction was so harsh that she decided to take a break from the spotlight.[19] In an interview with *InStyle* magazine in 2019 she admitted that she had spoken "too early," saying that "I think there was still a stigma around sharing so much truth, and it kind of got seen as me being self-indulgent or trying to gain attention."[20] Something her interviewer describes as "Snow was speaking out about mental health and pulling back the curtain on a deeply personal experience during a time when society was much less receptive to conversations about mental illness."[21] This reflects not only an awareness in the media in 2019 about mental health issues and how to write about them, but also an idea of the media at large as now being more responsible than it used to be in regard to these topics. Rather than engage in sensationalist coverage of breakdowns and trainwrecks, celebrity reporting assumed a more careful approach to issues of mental illness, indirectly informed by discourses of mental health awareness and advocacy. The increase in conversations around mental illness in popular media like *Cosmopolitan* and *Teen Vogue*, and among celebrities, served to normalize issues like depression and anxiety. One can imagine that portraying a suffering celebrity as an outrageous trainwreck became less appealing, as it in the process of normalization also is assumed that stars and regular people alike are afflicted by the issues. Portraying stars who live with mental illness as something to be shocked by (as the sensationalist trainwreck coverage does) assumes that the reader cannot relate to what the celebrity is going through and positions the audience at a distance, gawking at the spectacle of a famous person breaking down. When mental illnesses instead are considered common and something that can affect everyone, the coverage of celebrities going through such things takes a relatable approach that serves to present the famous person as "just like us" in their suffering. This is also indicative of a larger shift toward more ordinariness in celebrity branding and reporting, something propelled by the prevalence of social media, which I discuss further below.

I would also argue that this shift in approach to mental illness, specifically the tendency of celebrities themselves to speak in first person about their struggles, played a large part in mobilizing the #FreeBritney-movement that ultimately led to the dissolution of her conservatorship. The fan-led movement called attention to the wellbeing of Britney Spears under the conservatorship controlled by her father, in which the majority of her life was under his command and decision-making.[22] The image of Britney accessible to her fans was largely mediated through Instagram, which from 2015 and on became a minor cultural phenomenon, leading to the start of a podcast dedicated solely to interpreting the singer's activity on the platform.[23] At a time when other stars provided firsthand accounts of past troubles and ongoing diagnoses, Britney posted low-res selfies, inspirational quotes, and videos of herself dancing at the same spot in her house, with very little seemingly real info about what was going on in her life. The fans knew she had had a breakdown and then been placed under the conservatorship, but at no point had she herself sat down for a first-person confessional interview, or even produced a social media post in that vein, which in a media landscape ripe with those kinds of confessions stood out. I contend that the discrepancy between the way Britney's mental health was mediated and the prevalence of celebrity talk about mental illness——in the sense that her psychic wellbeing was NOT directly addressed at a time when this was a popular topic in celebrity media—— contributed to the success of the #FreeBritney-movement and the ultimate dissolution of her conservatorship in November 2021.[24]

It is also important to note that celebrities suffering from mental illnesses is not a new phenomenon. In the early modern and romantic period, madness was a sign of the melancholy philosopher-artist and of the genius of the Byronic iconoclastic artist.[25] The connection between

mental distress and creativity and talent continued into the twentieth century,[26] and at the start of the twenty-first century, "psychic turmoil is [still]
taken as a sign of artistic authenticity."[27] Often "suffering, dysfunction or
the personal flaw, once concealed but now revealed to the public" are just
as important elements to the celebrity story as high achievement.[28] Stories
about stars who "make it through" often encourage values of individual
autonomy and self-mastery[29] and end up reinforcing "neoliberal ideologies of meritocracy and competitive individualism."[30] But narratives of
celebrities struggling with mental illnesses have tended to be heavily gendered, working mostly in the favor of male stars. Nina K. Martin notes
that the breakdowns of male celebrities often are considered "fascinating,
demonstrating behavior that shores up stereotypical hetero-masculinity
(promiscuity and cheating, aggression and rage, linked with drugs and
alcoholism)."[31] Overcoming scandal in this context is a sign of heroism,
while "women's attempts to overcome their foibles are viewed as signifiers
of tragic instability and madness."[32] Gaston Franssen points out that the
same "ideology of competitive individualism" is at play for both male and
female breakdowns, but "with clear gendered differences: psychological
instability for male artists is associated with perseverance, credibility and
authenticity; for female artists, mental breakdown is seen as a sign of failure, inherent instability or a lack of resilience."[33]

Franssen analyzes Demi Lovato's celebrity health narrative and argues
that it is an exceptional story within the traditionally gendered discourses
mentioned above, because the star has managed to incorporate mental
distress into their brand in a way that has "ensured that she is perceived as
a self-confident artist and a successful entrepreneur of self-care."[34] I will
return to Franssen's analysis of Lovato below and build upon that with my
own. I argue that Lovato's story (of repeated breakdown, recovery, and
reinvention) is becoming less exceptional and more common among
female* stars. Stories of trauma and difficulties serve to make celebrities
more authentic and relatable, exemplifying a profitable vulnerability where
difficult subjects become integral to the star brand.

A CHANGING CELEBRITY MEDIA LANDSCAPE

It is also worth noting how celebrity reporting itself has changed throughout the 2010s and the role of social media in its evolvement. In 2008
celebrity journalism was dominated by blogs like *Perez Hilton* and *TMZ*,
which were ready to publish the most sensationalist stories, with little

concern over how it would affect the stars themselves. Celebrity scholar Anne Helen Petersen has described how celebrities experienced this as being (almost) completely out of control, with paparazzi willing to step over dead bodies to get valuable photos of their subjects (a spate of car crashes involving photographers and celebrities underscored this sentiment).[35] As the 2010s progressed, however, stars learned to utilize their own social media channels to circumvent the control of the paparazzi and the unscrupulous gossip blogs. Toward the end of the decade traditional outlets were reporting on what the stars were doing on social media, creating stories based on celebrities' Instagram posts and tweets.[36]

This goes hand in hand with Marwick and boyd's analysis of celebrity practice on Twitter, which they argue takes place through "the appearance and performance of 'backstage' access."[37] They conceptualize celebrity as "an organic and ever-changing *performative practice*" which involves "ongoing maintenance of a fan base, performed intimacy, authenticity and access, and construction of a consumable persona."[38] "Micro-celebrities," individuals who have built up a devoted audience on digital platforms, are pioneers and masters of this practice, but other kinds of celebrities have come to adopt the same methods to maintain their fanbases with the rise of social media.

The performed intimacy is especially important for my discussion here, and Marwick and boyd argue that celebrities reveal seemingly personal information on Twitter to establish "a sense of intimacy between participant and follower."[39] Heather Nunn and Anita Biressi argue similarly that an "'ideology of intimacy' has formed the conditions in which the celebrity, along with other public figures and the ordinary person, now labour as emotional subjects in the public arena."[40]

Since Marwick and boyd's 2011 article and Nunn and Biressi's 2010 piece, this way of practicing celebrity has only become more established and takes place not only on Twitter but also on Instagram and other social media platforms. Barker, Gill, and Harvey also argue that "we live in a world *suffused and saturated with representations of intimate relationships*."[41] Even though their examination of mediated intimacy primarily concerns romantic relationships and sex, the point about the domineering presence of intimate relationships carries over to issues like mental health, in that it explains the naturalness with which details of previously "personal" and "private" topics are now discussed out in the open.

DEFINING CELEBRITY

Another important aspect to keep in mind when discussing celebrity is its role as an economic condition that produces value and profit, and that involves a range of practices beyond the celebrity's professional employment (i.e. as musician or actor for example). During the first part of the twentieth century, the primary value of the Hollywood celebrity was to differentiate film products and generate attention for a film, but as the studio system collapsed and the entertainment business grew, a whole industry emerged that "found ways to generate value from the celebrity's whole life on and off the screen, creating lifestyle synergies between stars, products, services and events."[42]

The monetary value of the celebrity has always been dependent on the audience that it can deliver. Alison Hearn and Stephanie Schoenhoff examine how celebrity has changed as the measurements of audiences have become more and more specified. Various tools have been used to measure audience engagement, from the Nielsen ratings of television viewership, the Q score that measures familiarity and likeability, and the Klout score which claimed to measure and score the totality of a person's social media impact. Originally, the value a celebrity was able to generate came from box office and record sales. Eventually it moved into a larger field of endorsed products and direct marketing of their own commodities. For example, instead of endorsing or appearing in an ad for a perfume, celebrities began producing their own perfumes (or other wares) for direct sale to audiences, something that became common in the 1990s when celebrities "began to configure themselves explicitly as brands."[43] Within celebrity branding, the process of value generation is strengthened "because it relies so completely on the ongoing and infinitely malleable distinctiveness of the celebrity's 'personal' lifestyle."[44] Here authenticity becomes one of the most important elements determining the value of a celebrity, "beyond the roles played or music created, today's celebrity brand is predicated on convincing consumers of the authenticity of their inherent 'being' beyond the limelight."[45] This emphasis on authenticity is only heightened when it comes to micro-celebrities and influencers, for whom the "promise of authenticity" is a central aspect of their strong relation to their followers, the strength of which is what determines how much monetary value is invested in them by marketers and advertising agencies.[46] In other words, the increased intimacy between celebrities and fans is closely tied to a longer history of monetizing the celebrity's whole life by presenting a "real" image.

The "relatability" of *Cosmopolitan*'s mental health coverage, which manages to touch on difficult subjects but does so in a non-threatening and distanced way, fits well into this marketable authenticity. One can presume that a celebrity would want to appear real to convey authenticity and intimacy, but they would not want to do so in a way that presents too much difficulty or pain, because doing so might risk the audience/fan becoming uncomfortable and no longer acting as a consumer of whatever product is being sold in conjunction with the celebrity brand. The audience/fan still has to act as a consumer and generate monetary value, but they might be deterred from doing so if they get too sad or down from hearing about a celebrity's personal struggle. By presenting difficulties in distanced and relatable ways a celebrity can appear authentic without becoming "too much."[47]

Additionally, whether or not a social relationship is perceived as authentic or real is often determined based on the strength of the "commitment to the 'inner psychological concerns of each person.'"[48] The media discourse in which celebrities share their own experiences of depression and anxiety is thus one where fans are expecting greater personal connection to their idols. This creates a context for celebrity practice where disclosing private details is not out of the ordinary, but instead part of the norm. For celebrities, telling the world that you have suffered through depression might no longer be something that taints your image, but in fact improves it by contributing to the authenticity of your performance of self. As such, disclosing details about one's mental health might even be a strategical choice in order to maintain a close relationship with fans. When looking at the relationship between celebrity and fan in purely economic terms, the incorporation of vulnerability into the public narrative of the star becomes a profitable choice.

The tendency to share issues of mental health is also seen in the world of micro-celebrities, where several of the biggest stars in the world of beauty and lifestyle YouTubers have spoken openly and repeatedly about their struggles with anxiety.[49] Despite the still dominant perception of social media as "an archive of endlessly positive self-documentation," among micro-celebrities on sites like YouTube the display of negative affect is increasingly common.[50] Rachel Berryman and Misha Kavka present several examples of crying and anxiety vlogs made by YouTubers with large followings and argue that the displays of negative affects here become productive, in that they "cement authenticity, offer (self-)therapy and strengthen ties of intimacy between YouTubers and their followers."[51] An unfiltered and "raw" video of someone crying becomes in this context a sign of realness and vulnerability that reinforces the bonds between micro-celebrity and fan. In relation to the more traditional celebrities I discuss in this chapter, the continued success of micro-celebrities on platforms like YouTube influences the way that more traditional celebrities come to construct their own celebrity image. This includes a heightened (in comparison to previous eras) intimacy between celebrity and fans, that expresses itself in things like more openness about mental health struggles.

Lastly, this shift to more and more intimate channels of communication between celebrity and fans is also part of a turn toward ordinariness in celebrity culture. Joshua Gamson notes that the celebrity narrative that positions the famous as ordinary and "just like us" has long been used to make celebrities more relatable and invite identification with them.[52] The elevation of the ordinary has intensified from the 1990s and onwards, first with the rise of reality TV and its practice of making stars out of ordinary people, and then with the Internet and the possibility to become famous without the traditional celebrity industry.[53] This has only intensified with the rise of self-branding and the emergence of the social media influencer.[54]

Spotlight on Pop Stars

Both Demi Lovato and Selena Gomez have been prominent mental health advocates that have appeared frequently in my celebrity archive. I chose to focus on the two of them in this chapter because they have spoken about their issues repeatedly in very visible ways. Both of them were also child stars who made their debut on the children's show *Barney and Friends* (1992-2009). After getting to know each other on the television series, Lovato and Gomez developed a close friendship that became highly publicized——shown on magazine covers, in a series of homemade YouTube videos by the two stars, the made-for-TV-movie *Princess Protection Program*, and several unauthorized biographies about the "BFFs" (best friends forever).[55]

As girls and teen celebrities, Lovato and Gomez were at the center of US media culture's fascination with girls in the early 2000s. As Anita Harris argues, the girls seen in popular media tend to be either "can-do" girls who are confident and have almost infinite capacity for success, or "at-risk" girls who lack self-esteem and engage in risky behavior.[56] Both of these figures circulate together in media culture as examples to follow—— where the at-risk girl functions as a warning to the can-do girl, reminding her "that failure is an ever-lurking possibility that must be staved off through sustained application."[57] These two tropes come together in the above mentioned figure of the female trainwreck, a phenomenon Sarah Projansky in her work on girls in media culture calls the "'crash-and-burn' girl."[58] This is the girl who "has it all, but who—through weakness and/ or the inability to live with the pressure of celebrity during the process of growing up—makes a mistake and therefore faces a spectacular descent into at-risk status."[59] In her study of spectacular girls, Projansky puts Lovato in the fold of the "crash-and-burn" girl who had potential but fell into at-risk-status when she was involved in a scandal and subsequently went to rehab (more on that below). Gomez, on the other hand, is defined as a "super can-do girl" who is glamorous but playful and "the kind of girl anyone would want to be around."[60]

What becomes interesting for this book and the larger discussion of mediated representations of mental illness is that Lovato since their 2010 breakdown and revelation of a bipolar diagnosis, eating disorder and substance abuse has made several comebacks and has managed to successfully incorporate their mental distresses into the Demi Lovato brand in a way that recasts them as a "can-do girl" again. And Gomez has since 2016 been open about her struggles with depression and anxiety, effectively folding those into her image, including in the marketing of her own line of makeup which professes to promote mental wellbeing and has made mental health awareness a cornerstone of its brand.[61] Both Lovato and Gomez have successfully incorporated their mental struggles into their celebrity brands in ways that disrupt the "can-do—at-risk"—binary.

Lovato is an example of someone who first spoke out about their issues earlier in the decade, at a time when it was not as common for (especially female*) celebrities to be outspoken about mental illnesses. Their tell-all documentaries, many statements, and engagements with mental health advocacy have provided a rich archive from which to study how attitudes about mental health have taken shape during the 2010s. Gomez, who has only been open about her struggles since 2016, is instead an example of the mid-2010s openness around mental health issues, and her statements around them reveal the state of the more recent and mental-illness-aware media culture.

In addition to both having been very visible around issues of mental health, their positions in girl culture as crash-and-burn and can-do girls* respectively make their stories illustrative of how a postfeminist media culture that urges girls and women to be confident and empowered grapples with issues of mental illness.[62] In the discussion that follows I intend to show how Lovato and Gomez's celebrity health narratives, and the numerous confessions from female stars about their own mental health issues from 2015 and onwards, seem to suggest that the ideal postfeminist and neoliberal subject who works on herself constantly to achieve success has some room for failure as long as it is successfully overcome. In this sense the narratives I discuss here are of the same type that Shani Orgad and Rosalind Gill discuss in relation to the confidence cult of contemporary women's media, where failure is accepted "under the condition that it has been overcome."[63] A certain kind of anti-self-help book, where failure is celebrated, has become popular. But Orgad and Gill show how failure is only allowed when it has already been defeated, when it "can be referred to as something that happened and is safely sealed in the past."[64] The representation of emotional distress that we see here is thus one that involves a certain kind of distance to the problems at hand, rather than a depiction of the breakdown as it happens. In this sense these narratives also fit into what Angela McRobbie defines as a common trope of late-capitalist media culture: the perfect-imperfect-resilience.[65] For McRobbie, the perfect encourages women "to succeed meritocratically, while simultaneously introducing heightened competition, constantly redifferentiating and establishing division."[66] The imperfect then allows for some expressions of failure and critique of the impossibility of constant success, but it is quickly followed by resilience, which functions as a "bounce-back" mechanism that reinvigorates the aim for the perfect. My argument follows Orgad and Gill and McRobbie, and I contend that Lovato and Gomez present their struggles in a way that exemplifies profitable vulnerability——that is, their ailments add authenticity and relatability to their celebrity brands in profitable ways.

DEMI LOVATO: TROUBLED STAR AND EXPERT OF RE-INVENTION

Demi Lovato started their career in 2002, at the age of 10, on the children's television show *Barney and Friends* and had their breakthrough in the Disney Channel musical television film *Camp Rock* (2008) and its sequel *Camp Rock 2: The Final Jam* (2010). In addition to their television work, Lovato has released seven studio albums: *Don't Forget* (2008), *Here We Go Again* (2009), *Unbroken* (2011), *Demi* (2013), *Confident* (2015),

Tell Me You Love Me (2017) and *Dancing with the Devil... the Art of Starting Over* (2021). In early 2022, the singer's net worth was reportedly about $40 million.[67] In other words, their artistry is a big business involving a lot of money and employing a big team.

Lovato rose to fame at the age of 16 after starring in the Disney production *Camp Rock*, leading them to go on tour with the, at the time very popular, boy band the Jonas Brothers, who were also associated with the film and its sequel. In October 2010, after a performance in Columbia, Lovato punched one of their backup dancers and abruptly left the tour to go straight to rehab in Illinois. At the time it was reported that they were seeking treatment for "emotional and physical issues."[68] In April the following year, three months after leaving the treatment center, Lovato revealed in an interview with *People* magazine that, after seeking care for an eating disorder and self-harm, they had also received a bipolar disorder diagnosis.[69] In the trajectory of a celebrity breakdown, the tabloid press often sets the stage for how the audience will respond to the scandal, but the stars themselves have the power to talk back and confess or deny rumors.[70] Franssen notes that Lovato went far beyond merely salvaging their reputation, instead they embraced their "mental struggle and diagnosis with bipolar disorder and incorporated them into [their] celebrity narrative."[71] Barely a year after revealing their diagnosis, in March 2012, the documentary *Demi Lovato: Stay Strong* was released on MTV.[72] Here Lovato's fans got to follow the star as they prepared for and subsequently went on the *Unbroken* tour, to promote their newly released album. The documentary features several long interviews with Lovato and presents them as a star that has hit rock bottom but has come out stronger on the other side. The image used to promote it, which also frames its commercial breaks, shows the inside of Lovato's wrists, one of which has "stay" and the other "strong" tattooed on them. The film focuses mostly on the singer's eating disorder and self-harm behavior, and also mentions the bipolar diagnosis they received while in treatment.

Franssen's analysis of Lovato's celebrity health narrative focuses primarily on this 2012 documentary. He compellingly identifies three levels on which Lovato's recovery is narrativized in the film: "it entails a narrative of private struggle, which authenticates her crisis; a narrative of diagnosis, which reifies and externalizes the cause of her breakdown; and a narrative of self-improvement and self-transformation, which recalibrates her celebrity image."[73] I will return to these levels in my analysis of Lovato's second tell-all documentary, *Simply Complicated*.

Stay Strong also features several interviews with Lovato's fans before and after concerts. They talk about how they are inspired by the singer's honesty about their struggles and express a sentiment of "If Demi can do it so can I." One fan says "When Demi came out about her issues and about the cutting and the eating disorders I was just really inspired and that's why I told my parents about it and that's why I went to treatment," exemplifying the power of a celebrity telling their story. In this framing Lovato's mental distress and the willingness to speak openly about it becomes a "positive" aspect of their story, in that it is doing "good work" by inspiring others to get better. This is reflected in a scene where Lovato is seen leading their team in prayer before the start of a show. Here they not only express the hope that "we do our best performance possible," but also request God to "take whatever pain is inside these audience members [and] let them have fun tonight." In another scene Lovato is shown performing as their voiceover says "I wasn't given this voice just to sing" but that "there is a bigger picture and that is to use your voice, inspire people and to get people through their day and problems and to pick people up when they are down." Lovato's honesty about their struggles becomes a lifeline to their fans, who through Lovato can acknowledge their own problems.

A few others speak about how inspired they are by Lovato's show of strength and confidence, echoing the confidence cult(ure) described by Gill and Orgad and foreshadowing Lovato's 2015 album titled simply *Confident*.[74] The documentary being titled *Stay Strong*, the name of the tour featured in the film being *Unbroken*, and the subsequent album being titled *Confident*, all reinforce the focus of much popular media culture at the time to encourage women to be strong, empowered, and in charge. And the narrative of Lovato having had a break-down and then recovered fits well into the logic of confidence culture, where the presence of an already overcome vulnerability serves to make the confident subject more relatable.[75] And as Lovato's career goes on, they mobilize this already-dealt-with vulnerability over and over again, in distinctively profitable ways.

From Crash-and-Burn to Can-Do

In her analysis of three British female celebrities who had been labeled "bad girls" during the 1990s and early 2000s, Emma Bell argues that they used disclosures of mental illness to remove the "bad" label.[76] According to her, "after a period of media antagonism (and subsequent cultural and market devaluation), 'bad girl' celebrities can re-gain public attention and cultural value through revelations of mental illness."[77] The stars that Bell looks at ("Spice Girl Geri Halliwell, "ladette" Gail Porter, and "wild child" Kerry Katona) gained their original fame in the 1990s as part of the "Girl Power" and "ladette" wave in British popular culture at the time.[78] Their disclosures of mental illness happened in the late 1990s and early 2000s (and were thus not within the scope of my archive here) through autobiographical reality and life products such as memoirs and reality television shows, and were framed as repudiations of the pop-feminism associated with their original claims to fame. Bell describes how the confessions did give these women renewed attention and another shot at stardom, but they were often accompanied by derisions from both tabloid press and serious media. She concludes that "the cultural interest in these women depends on their being simultaneously in and out of control with regard to the circulation and contours of their public images," where their attempts at regaining control of their public images through mental illness revelations were derided and ridiculed in the media.[79] This makes the celebrities Bell studies different from the cases I have examined, where the stars have largely managed to maintain control over their health narratives. The discrepancies can be attributed both to the variation of national context (I focus on a US context and the British tabloids tend to be more ruthless in their celebrity coverage than American ones) and a shift in the mid-2010s toward more acceptance toward mental health awareness.

Nevertheless, what Lovato does in the 2012 documentary *Stay Strong* could be read through the lens that Bell describes. The move to put out their own account of the "breakdown" and rehab-stay can be seen as a way to take control over the public narrative about their personal life so as not to be labeled a "bad girl." By coming out and talking about their struggles, Lovato sidesteps outsider speculations about what may have caused their distress. This documentary also functions as a useful tool for Lovato to step away from the wholesome branding of the Disney channel that was their original claim to fame, and frame the launch of the album *Unbroken* (2011) with which they are shown touring in the film. This album has a more mature, grown-up, RnB-vibe compared to the singer's previous two albums which were in a more pop-rock vein (something Lovato discusses in the accompanying audio commentary to *Unbroken*). The revelation of mental illness struggles serves to cement Lovato's authenticity as a "real" person behind the wholesomeness of the Disney brand. The title of the album, *Unbroken*, quite literally reflects the "can-do girl" trope of confidence, resilience, and independence.[80] It is almost as if Lovato's team produced the *Stay Strong* documentary to clean up their image and re-do it as a "can-do woman" whose experiences only add to their appeal of strength and confidence. Something that Franssen picks up on in his analysis of the documentary, which he describes as "a representation *as well as* a performance of a process of self-management, producing an updated, better 'self' for Lovato."[81] This leads to the successful incorporation of their "crash-and-burn" status into a "can-do" narrative, something that the star will do multiple times again with a second documentary, subsequent relapse, and a third documentary.

In the years following the release of *Stay Strong* Lovato kept working and releasing albums at the same time as they established themselves as a mental health advocate. This included things like establishing a scholarship program in the name of their late father to help people pay for treatment at the CAST Recovery center where Lovato had gotten support, and releasing a book of affirmations (*Staying Strong: 365 Days a Year*, 2013) that reached the number one spot in the "Advice, How-to & Miscellaneous"-category of the New York Times bestseller list and was then followed by a companion book (*Staying Strong: A Journal*, 2014).[82] These two books and their success reveal how Lovato and their team managed to fold their painful experiences into the Lovato-brand, further authenticate their struggles, and quite literally profit off of them in book sales. In 2014 Lovato also embarked on the "Mental Health Listening and Engagement Tour," sponsored by a pharmaceutical company and a few mental health organizations.[83] In 2016 they announced that they would host seminars with fans to discuss mental health issues as part of their tour; then appeared at the Democratic National Convention to give a speech about mental health in conjunction with endorsing Hillary Clinton; and in September they revealed in an interview with CBS that they co-owns part of the rehab center where they received treatment.[84] These are only a few of the many actions taken by Lovato during these years to establish their brand as a mental health advocate. The ease with which this aspect is folded into their celebrity brand shows the profitability of mobilizing vulnerability in this way.

Simply Complicated

In October 2017 Lovato released their second "tell-all" documentary, *Demi Lovato: Simply Complicated*, to coincide with the release of the album *Tell Me You Love Me*, this time on YouTube.[85] The fact that Lovato chose to release their second autobiographical documentary on this platform rather than a traditional distributor shows the leverage of YouTube as a media actor but also the influence of the microcelebrity vloggers who have made the platform what it is today. *Stay Strong* was released on MTV in 2012 and is not freely available anywhere online. *Simply Complicated*, on the other hand, is still available worldwide on YouTube, making this version of Lovato's celebrity health narrative as accessible to fans as the videos of native YouTube stars.

This documentary starts with Lovato stating: "I actually had anxiety around this interview .... because the last time I did an interview this long I was on cocaine," referring to the 2012 *Stay Strong* documentary. This sets the stage for this newer film to be "rawer" and more "real" than the previous one, which is supported by Lovato's repeated confessions of manipulating those around them and saying "I wasn't working my program. I wasn't ready to get sober. I was sneaking it on planes, sneaking it in bathrooms, sneaking it throughout the night."

Lovato and their team re-tell the story of the initial breakdown that happened on tour with the Jonas Brothers in more detail than in the earlier documentary and with input from the Jonas Brothers themselves. Their manager, Phil McIntyre, is also featured speaking extensively about the darkness beneath the surface of Lovato's life during 2012 and 2013, while they were telling the world that they were sober and healed. The life coach Mike Bayer (author of several self-help books and an expert contributor to the Dr Phil television show), who is one of the founders of the CAST-treatment centers and who was hired by McIntyre to help Lovato get out of addiction, is also interviewed in this documentary. McIntyre, Bayer, and Lovato speak at length about how difficult Lovato was to work with during their darkest days, and they all describe the moment when it came to a breaking point. McIntyre, the manager, recounts how he had gotten Lovato's entire team onboard to stage a kind of intervention, where they told the singer that if they did not commit to getting better, he and the entire team would leave. Lovato responded by crying and asking what they could do, and Bayer tells them to hand over their cellphone. In a montage of McIntyre and Bayer recounting the event, they describe how Lovato smashed their phone and then put it in a glass of water to finalize its destruction. As he is holding Lovato's old phone, McIntyre says "this was the gateway to everything, this was the wrong people, it was drug dealers, it was a lot of the negative influences in her life were coming through the cellphone." And as if to emphasize that this was not Lovato being forced to give up their autonomy, the singer comments next that "I think that approached worked for me because, it sounds silly but it was the beginning of the process of surrendering. At the end of the day it was my decision." Next, Bayer and McIntyre describe the bizarre circumstances of Lovato's life at the time, when the star was serving as a judge on the reality television program *X-factor*. Bayer says "Meanwhile she's a judge on *X-factor*. She's 19 years old and she's in her first year of sobriety." McIntyre continues: "What nobody knows is that while she was a judge she's living in a sober apartment, with roommates, she's having to do chores, she has no cellphone. She is completely and totally submitted to the process of recovery." Next Lovato says: "You really have to lean into the people who are trying to support you. Like my family, like Mike [Bayer] and Phil [McIntyre]. You know you really have to surrender because that's when the change is gonna happen." Notably, none of them says anything about why Lovato had to work as a judge on *X-factor* while going through recovery, or why they had to keep churning out albums when they were suffering.

This particular storytelling montage is thrilling for someone interested in Lovato's personal life, by telling viewers what it was "actually" like during those years they are invited into the symbolical backstage of their life. In giving fans access to this previously closed-off part of Lovato's life, the documentary engages in the "performative practice" of an effective celebrity narrative.[86]

In many ways *Simply Complicated* is a complex and multifaceted portrayal of living with bipolar disorder, addiction, and an eating disorder. Lovato reveals to their manager on camera that they had a relapse with their eating disorder related to the recent breakup with their boyfriend of many years. This together with the conversations about how hard it was for them to get sober, paints a picture of recovery and living with mental illness as an ongoing work in progress, something one has to keep working at for the rest of one's life. This follows the logic of much mental health and addiction advocacy, but it also fits very well into the project of neoliberal and postfeminist subjectivity, where the subject has to continually work on herself to constantly better herself.[87] And for all of Lovato's and their team's honesty about their struggles, what is left glaringly untouched is why they had to keep working while they were in such a vulnerable place. Following the logic of postfeminism and neoliberalism, the documentary seems to suggest that it is ok to struggle with things like addiction, eating disorders and mental illness, as long as you keep working against these difficulties and keep producing new things and adding to the labor market. The logic at work in Lovato's treatment program also reflects Scharff and Gill's observations about the "psychic life" of neoliberalism and postfeminism, where you have to work at bettering not only your career or physical body but also your affects.[88]

The same levels of narrativization found in the previous documentary, *Stay Strong*, are present in *Simply Complicated*. There is "a narrative of private struggle, which authenticates her crisis."[89] Interestingly, most of the private struggles presented in the later film invalidate the authenticity and "realness" of what was presented in the earlier one. This is most starkly exemplified in Lovato's opening statement in the second film about using cocaine while filming the first one. But this is not presented as something that invalidates the truth and authenticity conveyed by Lovato, rather it serves to reinforce their realness in portraying them as extraordinarily bold in their current honesty.

Also folded into the narrative of the singer's private struggle in the second film is the pressure under which they were under while working for Disney, touring, and recording an album all at the same time. The fact that Lovato was bullied in school is also mentioned as the cause of their troubles, as is the dysfunctional relationship with their biological father, who is described as an "addict and alcoholic." But it is the revelation of the bipolar diagnosis that ties it all together, working here as it did in the first documentary to reify and externalize the cause of her issues.[90] At about 20 minutes into the film, just after having recounted the violent incident while on tour in Columbia, another member of Lovato's team, John Taylor, says "that was when it dawned on me that this was probably a much bigger situation than just a kid who wanted to party." The "much bigger situation" is implied to be the bipolar diagnosis, which Lovato's manager recounts them getting in the following scene. Next, the singer explains it as follows:

> When I got diagnosed with bipolar disorder, it just made sense. When I was younger I didn't know why I would stay up so late writing and playing music. And then I learned about episodes of mania and I realized that that's probably what it was—I was manic. In a way I knew that it wasn't my fault anymore. Something was actually off with me.

Here a connection is made between the bipolar diagnosis and Lovato's creativity, which reflects the reverence in American culture for mania that

Emily Martin identified in her comprehensive study of bipolar disorder in the US.[91] This is echoed in Franssen's (2020) analysis of Lovato's celebrity health narrative, in which he identifies the bipolar diagnosis specifically as fitting "within a broader, distinctly gendered 'spectacularization' of female breakdown and ongoing self-improvement."[92]

Lovato's description of the diagnosis as relieving them of fault echoes Eva Illouz's analysis of therapeutic narratives, which she argues makes the individual responsible for her psychic wellbeing, but does so by "removing any notion of moral fault."[93] Illouz contends that this kind of narrative "enables one to mobilize the cultural schemes and values of moral individualism, of change and self-improvement," but by "transposing these to childhood and to deficient families, one is exonerated from the weight of being at fault for living an unsatisfactory life."[94] We see that in the case of Lovato with their alcoholic father and the bullying from classmates, but also with the bipolar diagnosis. This suggests that in therapeutic narratives of the late 2010s, a mental illness diagnosis weighs just as much, if not more, than the dysfunctional family dynamics of the Freudian-dominated narratives of the twentieth century. By adding a medical diagnosis to the mix, Lovato is one step further removed from being at fault for their troubles than if it was "just" their dysfunctional father and bullying. But nevertheless, Lovato's condition is still something that needs to be continually managed, which is shown in the "recovery montage" toward the end of the film. It is also in this montage that the narrative of self-improvement and self-transformation that "recalibrates her celebrity image" is found.[95] This part of *Simply Complicated* is similar to the earlier documentary, but in this version it is amped up, with physical exercise taking center stage as a particular savior.

As the camera pans over a Los Angeles road lined with palm trees, Lovato's voice says "Everybody has their own path and recovery. For me it's about going to therapy, working my program, and having an honest relationship with myself and the other people around me." As the singer is shown working out, sparring with professional boxers and then practicing Jiu-Jitsu, their voice-over says "The gym really helps, and I know I would be in a very dark place without it." Then we see a montage of very well-lit shots of Lovato exercising to upbeat music as they say "I'm on a journey to discover what it's like to be free of all demons." During the gym sequence, Lovato's life coach Bayer explains how he introduced the star to Jiu-Jitsu specifically because it involves a "reward system that takes many many many years to get through," with the implied effect that they will be busy advancing within this kind of exercise for a long time to come. Exercise is a remedy commonly prescribed as part of mental illness treatment and it is not surprising that it is part of the singer's recovery plan. But it is remarkable how well this depiction of the role of exercise in Lovato's life fits with the neoliberal and postfeminist subject who never stops working on herself. Here the script about the benefits of working out is slightly new in that it is not (only) about getting a desirable body, but about keeping a distressed mind in check.

The last part of the documentary also expresses both a postfeminist and a popular feminist ethos, showing Lovato and their friends discussing dating. At one point the singer says "I'm on a dating app with both guys and girls. I am open to human connection whether that's through a male or a female that doesn't matter to me." Next Lovato's stylist helps them pick out a date outfit, which turns into a montage of the singer in sexy poses as they say "When I'm comfortable in my own skin I feel confident and when I feel confident I feel sexy and when I feel sexy, watch out." Then we see Lovato's friends talk about how fun "single Demi" is, to which the star responds "There's like a certain stigma around a woman having casual sex and for me I just feel like it's my body and it's my choice and it's exciting and it's a connection with somebody and it's fun." This sequence aligns Lovato with the popular feminism that Sarah Banet-Weiser identifies as a prevalent feature of contemporary media culture. The star is here positioned both as a desirable sexual subject who is up for anything (a postfeminist trope) and by pointing out the double standard for women having casual sex, they also politicize their actions (albeit in the most gentle ways) and aligns them with "feminist expressions and politics [that] are brandable [and] commensurate with market logics."[96] This is a kind of feminism "that focus[es] on the individual body ... [and] that emphasize[s] individual attributes such as confidence, self-esteem, and competence as particularly useful to neoliberal self-reliance and capitalist success."[97] The affective position expressed by Lovato here also echoes (again) the confidence cult described by Orgad and Gill, where individual achievement and self-esteem can solve structural issues.[98]

The notion of recovery as an ongoing process is different from the victim-to-victor narratives that Lisa Blackman describes, in which the journey to recovery starts by acknowledging the illness, followed by the adoption of a psychiatric treatment plan that ultimately cures the person afflicted so that they overcome the trouble once and for all.[99] What we see in the case of Lovato is instead a dedication to always be working at getting and staying better. This is a common aspect of addiction recovery, where the subject, masculine or feminine, is told that their condition will never end but can be eternally managed. What Lovato's case shows is how well this recovery narrative fits into the notion of the ideal neoliberal and postfeminist subject who constantly works on herself to improve herself at every turn. This is partly because the singer is recovering from not only substance abuse issues, but also an eating disorder and bipolar disorder, which opens up their health narrative for more than just "addicts" to identify with. Lovato's story celebrates and confirms a neoliberal ideology of meritocracy, where overcoming repeated crises and setbacks while remaining productive "even under the pressures of the media, the market and mental illness" positions them as "a shining example of the neoliberal, self-managing subject."[100] That Lovato as a female* celebrity is able to inhabit this position, where traditionally it has mostly been famous men who have been able to reinvent themselves after scandal (as discussed above), becomes less exceptional when one takes into account the feminist media studies work on women as ideal neoliberal subjects.[101] What Lovato's celebrity health narrative and the numerous confessions from female stars about their own mental health issues from 2015 and onwards seem to suggest, is that the ideal postfeminist and neoliberal subject who works on herself constantly to achieve success has some room for failure as long as it is successfully overcome. This, again, fits well into Orgad and Gill's analysis of a confidence culture in which vulnerability is allowed when it appears as something that is in the past.[102] By combining the process of addiction recovery with mental illness recovery, Lovato's narrative indirectly challenges the victim-to-victor narrative and reconfigures the idea of being completely cured of mental illness into one of more continual maintenance. This is on the one hand truer to how managing mental illness works for most people, but it also reveals that the presence of traumatic events is not a taint on a celebrity's image but rather an opportunity to strengthen the profitability of the celebrity brand through shared vulnerability.

The Public Acknowledgment of a Relapse

That the process of recovery is never complete was seen for Lovato the year after *Simply Complicated* was released. On June 21, 2018, the singer released a single titled "Sober," which was introduced on Twitter as simply "My truth."[103] The lyrics seemed to suggest a relapse into substance abuse, with the chorus going "Mama, I'm so sorry I'm not sober any-more/ And daddy please forgive me for the drinks spilled on the floor/ To the ones who never left me, we've been down this road before/ I'm so sorry/ I'm not sober anymore."[104] A few days later it was reported that Lovato was in a feud with life coach Bayer and that every photo and mention of their name had been wiped from the website of the CAST-center that he runs and which Lovato had previously been a co-owner of.[105] And on July 24, a little over a month after the release of "Sober," Lovato was rushed to the hospital after an overdose that almost killed them.[106] About two weeks after the incident Lovato posted a note to their fans on Instagram, in which they said "I have always been transparent about my journey with addiction. What I've learned is that this illness is not something that disappears or fades with time. It is something I must continue to overcome and have not done yet."[107] Here again is the notion of addiction and mental illness as something that needs to be constantly worked at.

The release of "Sober" can on the one hand be read as an honest way of portraying the struggle of addiction and the very common experience of relapsing. But on the other hand, it can be seen as a way of incorporating Lovato's struggles into their brand and literally profiting off of them (Sober was certified Gold by The Recording Industry Association of America in August 2019).[108] Or a less cynical reading of the situation might be that the release of the single and the confession of their relapse was not, as might have been the case in other eras and with other artists, a taint on their brand but instead fit neatly into the larger "Lovato product" and almost functioned as confirmation of their authenticity.

Another thing to note in relation to Lovato's relapse is the outpouring of support from fans. A day after the report about the overdose, a fan account on Twitter started the hashtag #HowDemiHasHelpedMe, urging other fans to "share your stories and positive things so hopefully Demi sees positive things if she comes online."[109] The hashtag was trending on Twitter as fans began posting their stories and it was covered by several media outlets.[110] One notable example of a fan contribution was the following:

> The night I attempted suicide Demi had a performance on tv. My dad was watching it and not me. I was upstairs in my room taking pills to overdose. I heard [Lovato's song] skyscraper from my room so I told my mom I took pills and checked into a hospital for 8 Days.[111]

Other fans have responded to this tweet with things like "You are so strong! I hope you are better now," "So glad that you are still here," and "I'm sending you a long tight hug. Thank you for sharing your story."[112] Like this the fans show support not just for Lovato, but also for each other.

The reciprocal acts by the fans in sharing how Lovato has helped them might be a way to help each other through the public display of vulnerability on social media, something I discuss more in the following chapter. Because even if they purport to write to Lovato, the immediate audience is not the singer themselves (the assumption on social media is that stars usually do not read everything that is said about them, exemplified in what an occasion it is for fans when they do get a response from their idol), but other fans. In this way the outpouring of support for the celebrity becomes in itself a forum for sharing experiences and making each other feel less alone.

Another example of the outpouring of support from Lovato's fans at the time was a group of fans gathering in Atlantic City on the night when the singer was supposed to perform but had canceled due to the overdose. A group of over 60 "Lovatics" (what their fans call themselves) gathered to sing their songs together to show their support for the singer. One fan wrote on Twitter about the gathering: "Omg the people in Atlantic City for the Demi tribute are in a circle talking about how Demi has helped them and some of them even started crying :(the bond we have over Demi is so special."[113] Here Lovato's openness about their issues becomes a way for fans to share their own experiences with each other and get support.

Since the 2018 relapse Lovato has made a large-scale comeback, first at the 2020 Grammys with a performance that was widely praised for its display of vulnerability.[114] In the spring of 2021 they released their third tell-all documentary (this time in the form of a four-part YouTube series) in conjunction with the release of a new album, both of which were titled *Dancing with the Devil*.[115] In the docuseries Lovato and their team bare it all, revealing that the singer had been using heroin and crack cocaine, and that the overdose involved "aftermarket pills" laced with the extremely strong opioid Fentanyl that nearly killed them.[116] At the same time they released a music video that featured Lovato in a fictional reenactment of the overdose and the hospital stay that followed it.[117] In this way it is clear that the cyclical nature of Lovato's bipolar disorder and the always present risk of relapse into substance abuse or eating disorder are not the dire threats to their life and career as they might have been in previous eras. Instead, Lovato's struggles and their overcoming them serve to strengthen their brand as "pop's self-help princess."[118]

SELENA GOMEZ: CAN-DO GIRL TURNED MENTAL HEALTH ADVOCATE

Like Lovato, Selena Gomez had her acting debut on the children's show *Barney & Friends*, where she appeared during 2002–2004 from age 10 to 12. She then gained wider fame as the lead on the Disney channel show *Wizards of Waverly Place* (2007–2012) and subsequently starred in a multitude of films, some aimed at the Disney audience and others being more controversial, like Harmony Korine's *Spring Breakers* (2012) and Woody Allen's *A Rainy Day in New York* (2019). Beyond her acting work she has released three albums with her former band *Selena Gomez and the Scene: Kiss & Tell (2009), A Year Without Rain (2010),* and *When the Sun Goes Down (2011),* all of which attained gold certifications and reached the top ten in the US. She has also released three albums as a solo artist: *Stars Dance* (2013), *Revival* (2015), and *Rare* (2020), all of which debuted at number one in the US.[119] Additionally, she has executive produced the Netflix drama show *13 Reasons Why* (2017-2020) and the documentary series *Living Undocumented* (2019). In early 2022, Gomez's net worth is reportedly $75 million.[120] Gomez's brand is thus, like Lovato's, a big enterprise involving a lot of money and employing a large number of people.

As mentioned above, Gomez had an overall more wholesome persona than Lovato, staying away from the kind of scandal that the latter singer was involved in (even if Gomez was in an on-and-off relationship with fellow young artist Justin Bieber from 2010-2018 that led to a lot of speculations from fans and the media, those rumors were primarily about the state of their partnership).[121] In 2013 Gomez canceled the end of a planned tour to "spend some time" on herself, and in early 2014 she checked in to an Arizona rehab facility. This led to tabloid speculation about drug or alcohol abuse, but when she chose to speak about the events the following year she revealed that she had been diagnosed with the autoimmune disease lupus and had been receiving chemotherapy for it at the time.[122] It was not until in August 2016, also in relation to the cancelation of a planned tour, that she revealed that she was suffering from anxiety and depression. In a statement to *People* magazine, she said that she had "discovered that anxiety, panic attacks and depression can be side effects of lupus, which can present their own challenges." Adding, "I want to be proactive and focus on maintaining my health and happiness and have decided that the best way forward is to take some time off … I know I am not alone by sharing this, I hope others will be encouraged to address their own issues."[123] Here again the logic is that if Gomez with her large audience speaks out, it will inspire others to seek help. Additionally, in the *People* magazine story about the break a "source close to Gomez" tells the outlet that it is "'absolutely not related to alcohol or substance abuse' and was prompted after she 'hadn't felt like herself' over the last couple of months."[124] Here a clear demarcation is made against addiction issues, which indirectly serves to separate the anxiety and depression that Gomez was suffering from, from any assumption about the misuse of alcohol or drugs. This can be read as Gomez's team trying to deny rumors about her abusing substances and make clear that she is not like one of the many other starlets whose troubles are the result of too much partying (like in the case of many of the "trainwrecks" mentioned earlier). Even if addiction issues are increasingly considered to be a disease that is out of the control of the person suffering them, there is still a level of irresponsibility attached to the notion of someone getting addicted, as it presumes an engagement with illicit drugs or excessive amounts of alcohol at some point. By coming out as suffering from anxiety and depression as a result of her lupus, Gomez's issues are indirectly defined as rooted in a biomedical paradigm beyond her control.

A few months after initially announcing that she was taking a break to focus on her mental health, Gomez appeared at the American Music Awards (AMAs) in November 2016. In the acceptance speech for Best Female Artist in the Pop/Rock genre, the singer addressed the break, saying "I had everything and I was absolutely broken inside. And I kept it all together enough to never let you down, but I kept too much together, to where I let myself down." She thanked her fans for their loyalty during this time and added "if you are broken, you do not have to stay broken."[125] The speech at the AMAs was widely praised for its sincerity and honesty, with many media outlets pointing out that Gomez held back the tears while delivering it, as well as how other celebrities in attendance at the awards show seemed to appreciate what she was saying.[126]

After initially opening up about her mental health issues, Gomez repeatedly spoke out for mental illness awareness, prompting *Vogue* to describe her as "a compelling new voice for a generation of young women … [who is] breaking down conversational barriers surrounding emotional health" in March 2017. In this interview she mentions rehab, group therapy, and dialectical behavior therapy (DBT) as elements that have helped her, revealing that she sees her therapist five times a week.[127]

In a cover story for the September 2017 issue of *InStyle* magazine, titled "Selena Gomez Is Grown Up, in Love, and Taking Control of Her Mental Health," the journalist describes Gomez as having "a particularly potent power: Her celebrity comes not just from what she creates, how she looks, and whom she dates but from how she has suffered and how she has picked herself up."[128] In the interview accompanying the piece Gomez talks about her 90-day stay in a treatment center the previous year, how insecurity is something she works on in therapy, and how she is learning to stand up for herself. Here, just like in Lovato's health narrative, Gomez is portrayed as having successfully overcome, or rather as successfully managing, her mental health issues. The journalist's description of this experience as giving her "a particularly potent power" marks Gomez's suffering as something that adds to her celebrity and star power. That she has been to rehab is not a negative point on her resume; on the other hand, it seems to be a valuable experience that gives Gomez a maturity and frankness that only adds to the authenticity of her brand.

Just like with Lovato, Gomez's struggles were recurring. Later in 2017, it was revealed that she had a kidney transplant from a close friend and subsequently "laid low" for a while, not promoting her work or posting on social media. Then in January 2018 she checked into a "two-week wellness" program to regroup as a preventative measure for her mental health.[129] A few months later, she said in an interview in *Harper's Bazaar* that her struggle with depression and anxiety is "not something I feel I'll ever overcome" adding that "it's a battle I'm gonna have to face for the rest of my life, and I'm okay with that because I know that I'm choosing myself over anything else."[130] Here she reflects the notion of mental illness recovery as a constant struggle, as displayed also in Lovato's health narrative. Additionally, the phrase "choosing myself over anything else" fits well into a hyper-individualized neoliberal and postfeminist culture that positions the self as something to work on and prioritize at all costs.

The state of Gomez's mental health became a widely discussed topic again in the fall of 2018, first when she announced that she would be taking a social media break (at the time she was the most followed person on Instagram) and a few months later when she was reportedly hospitalized twice in two weeks with issues related to the kidney transplant.[131] These hospitalizations caused her to have an "emotional breakdown" which led to her checking into a mental health facility to receive DBT.[132] This breakdown was not portrayed, as it might have been in other eras, as a sign of "failure, inherent instability or a lack of resilience," but instead it was incorporated into her health narrative of struggle and maintenance of mental health.[133]

She then broke her silence in January of 2019 with a post on Instagram to reflect on the previous year, one "of self-reflection, challenges and growth."[134] In September 2019 Gomez received an award for furthering "the public's understanding of psychiatric illness and mental health" from the McLean Hospital, known for its psychiatric expertise and associated with Harvard Medical School.[135] In conjunction with accepting the award the singer also revealed that she herself had received treatment there for mental health issues, and in April 2020 she disclosed that while there she had received a bipolar diagnosis.[136][137]

This latter revelation happened not in an interview with a magazine or even on her own social media channels, but on the Instagram live talk show Bright Minded, hosted by fellow former child actor and musician Miley Cyrus during the initial COVID-19 lockdown.[138] The news was widely reported in multiple media outlets.[139] When asked why she had decided to tell the world about her diagnosis in this format instead of in a traditional interview, Gomez said that she "liked the rawness of the show" and felt comfortable to share her diagnosis with Cyrus because of the casual atmosphere.[140] This confirms the increased intimacy and ordinariness of contemporary celebrity and in their communication with fans.

Gomez has not done any big tell-all documentaries, like Lovato has. Instead the communication around her mental health happens in interviews, through her (and her peer's) social media channels, and indirectly in her work as an artist, which broaches mental illness and sadness in general.

Gomez was an executive producer of the Netflix show *13 Reasons Why* (2017-2020), which follows a high school in the aftermath of a student's suicide (and that was subject to heavy coverage by *Teen Vogue*). As mentioned in Chap. 3, the show became immensely popular with its target demographic but received harsh critique from suicide prevention organizations, teachers, and parents, who argued that it glorifies suicide and simplifies complex mental health issues.[141] The fact that Gomez has produced a television show that goes against the message of traditional mental illness awareness and suicide prevention organizations casts an interesting light on her advocacy for mental illness sufferers.

Additionally, in the Spotify music video for her May 2017 single "Bad Liar" Gomez portrays what can be called a "sad aesthetic."[142] The photo promoting the single shows Gomez lying down on a disheveled bed, staring at the viewer with a look full of sadness and hopelessness. Her hands are held together by a white silk rope, on one wrist she is wearing a yellow hospital bracelet spelling out the word "risk," and further up on the same arm a band-aid. Fans started speculating in the comments section on Gomez's Instagram about whether the bracelet and the band-aid were supposed to symbolize a suicide attempt. The photographer Petra Collins clarified (also on Instagram) that it had nothing to do with suicide, but that Gomez had come straight from a lupus-related hospital visit to the photo shoot.[143] Even if this is the real story behind the photograph, leaving the bracelet and the band-aid on results in an image that connotes self-harm and suicide for most people who do not know the back story. Interestingly, the above video is no longer available on Spotify and on Gomez's YouTube channel another, much lighter, video is listed as the official one for the song. The second, official version, takes place in a 1970s high school setting where Gomez plays several different characters in a family drama with unclear outcomes. An audio-only video of "Bad Liar" that has the still image from the above-described video as its background is still available, but the full moving image film is nowhere to be found on the star's YouTube or Spotify sites. This seems to be mostly due to the fact that the video with Spotify was an exclusive collaboration with that platform, but nevertheless it is notable that the more melancholic and self-destructive aspects of the first video are completely absent in the official one that remains available on the singer's channels.[144]

Playing with this self-harming aesthetic positions Gomez somewhat off-center of the "victim to victor" narrative and the idea of overcoming struggles through perseverance displayed in much of Lovato's celebrity health narrative. In interviews, she acknowledges that things like rehab and therapy have helped her, but then she nearly glorifies feeling bad in her work as an artist and TV producer. Here she is flirting with the "sad girl" aesthetic embraced by self-identified sad girls on sites like Tumblr and Instagram, which I will address further in the next chapter.[145]

Postfeminist Sadness

I want to mention artist Lana del Rey here as a means of understanding the trends that circulated on the music scene during the 2010s. The style of del Rey's music and visual representations is similar to the sad aesthetic that Gomez is experimenting with in some of her work. Del Rey, however, has not spoken about specific diagnoses like Lovato and Gomez, and she is absent from the compilation lists of celebrities speaking about mental illnesses. What she has spoken about is a period of heavy drinking in her early teens that led to her being sent to boarding school at age 14 and then getting sober at 18.[146] Instead of saying that she suffers from depression, anxiety, or any other established diagnosis, the singer has said that she thinks "ceaselessly of death" and that she has dealt with panic attacks but only attended therapy three times because she is "really most comfortable sitting in that chair in the studio, writing or singing."[147] And most notoriously, she said "I wish I was dead already" while citing Amy Winehouse and Kurt Cobain as her heroes, both of whom died at the age of 27.[148] Del Rey's official statements put her more in the role of having created a persona of being sad, rather than adopting the language of mental health advocacy in the way that Lovato and Gomez have.

Del Rey sings about female weakness and dependence in a way that makes it seem like she is enjoying it. These themes are present in much of her work (her first record having the apt title "Born to Die"), but is especially visible on her 2014 album "Ultraviolence" which is dominated by themes of submission and self-destructiveness in relation to various men. One line that particularly seems to encourage the abusive relationships portrayed throughout the album is a quote from a 1962 Carol King and Gerry Goffin song: "he hit me and it felt like a kiss," sung on the title track "Ultraviolence." The persona del Rey communicates on this record is one that takes melancholic pleasure in not getting what she wants and sometimes hints at deriving pleasure from abuse.

As discussed in Chap. 1, del Rey's 2011 debut provoked many by portraying a woman who did not know what she wanted in a popular music landscape filled with women brimming over with confidence and determination.[149] When she released "Ultraviolence" in 2014 she was critiqued as outright anti-feminist on the grounds of glorifying female weakness and dependency.[150] This was also around the same time as pop stars like Beyonce and Taylor Swift embraced a popular feminism that encourages female strength and independence. Del Rey's message of female weakness and dependence seemed to go directly counter to the strength advocated by popular feminism at the time.

In contrast, when Gomez spoke about her choice to be open about her depression and anxiety three years later, in 2017, she told *Vogue*: "We girls, we're taught to be almost too resilient, to be strong and sexy and cool and laid-back ... We also need to feel allowed to fall apart."[151] Here she speaks the language of (post)feminist empowerment, but instead of empowering women to be strong she wants to empower them to feel vulnerable. Something changed during the time between del Rey's emergence on the music scene and Gomez's call for girls to be vulnerable.

Scholars like Catherine Vigier noted already in 2012, when del Rey was a highly contested artist, that she gave "expression to some of the profound dissatisfactions that women continue to feel" despite having "followed mainstream society's prescriptions for success in what has been called a post-feminist world, but who find that real liberation and genuine satisfaction elude them."[152] During this time other celebrities expressed similar sentiments and were similarly contested. For example, Lena Dunham's show *Girls* premiered in 2012 and became the focus of many contested debates about whether or not the dysfunctional and dissatisfied characters she brought to the screen were feminist or not. Zoe Alderton makes an analysis of del Rey in relation to the critique of her as non-feminist, noting that she "represents narratives of female weakness, sadness, and failure" and "speaks to a generation who feel cut out of their forebears' market economy."[153] Alderton specifically states that the acknowledgment of weakness should not be something that hurts the feminist cause:

> Admitting that we are depressed or hurt should not make us less of a feminist. Natural human desires for those who hurt us, or for ill-conceived romances, should not make us feel as though we have betrayed our gender or let down the feminist cause.[154]

The sentiment Gomez expresses in her call for girls to be allowed to fall apart is the same as Alderton expresses here in relation to feminism. Even if Gomez does not name feminism directly, the reference to girls being asked to be "resilient ... strong and sexy and cool and laid-back"[155] reflects the demands of a popular feminism "that focus[es] on the individual body ... [and] that emphasize[s] individual attributes such as confidence, self-esteem, and competence as particularly useful to neoliberal self-reliance and capitalist success."[156] Both del Rey and Gomez, then, seem to respond to a media culture that demands overt positivity and confidence of young women.

Rather than suggest that either of them was the singular catalyst for more sadness in popular culture, I understand them both as giving expression to sentiments circulating in the shared culture and their success in delivering a certain message being dependent on the yearning of audiences to hear about those issues. These themes will be further explored in the next chapter, where I examine the figure of the sad girl, that in some iterations is closely tied to del Rey.

A 2019 analysis of del Rey's impact on music in conjunction with the release of her album *Norman Fucking Rockwell* credited the singer with making mainstream music more sad.[157] This is based not only on the writer's own observations (as is common in music journalism) but also on a 2018 study from researchers at the University of California at Irvine, which analyzed 500,000 popular songs released in the UK from 1985 to 2015 and classified them according to mood.[158] According to this research, there was "a clear downward trend in 'happiness' and 'brightness', as well as a slight upward trend in 'sadness,'" indicating that mainstream music has become statistically sadder.[159] This shift has only become more felt since then, with the artist Billie Eilish taking the world by storm with her sad and melancholic sound, winning five Grammys at the 2020 awards ceremony and composing the theme song for the 2021 Bond film.[160]

In the above mentioned analysis of del Rey's impact on music, Al Horner traces the roots of del Rey's sound to the niche music genre of "torch songs," defined as "a form of pop that is traditionally by and about downtrodden women who suffer at the hands of emotionally abusive men, but continue to love them devotionally anyways."[161] So while del Rey definitely did not invent this sad genre of music, she was instrumental in bringing it into the contemporary mainstream and use it to express "a very 21st-century sadness."[162] Horner also connects the shift toward a sad sound with the changed conversations around mental health and illness, stating that "in 2019, there's infinitely more room for discussions about depression in chart music than 10 years ago, mirroring wider social trends."[163] So even if Horner ascribes del Rey a lot of agency in making this happen, I do not necessarily think it was only del Rey who was driving this change, but rather that she was part of a wider social shift toward more sadness in popular culture, that came as a response to an overtly upbeat and empowerment focused feminine media culture.

The "sad aesthetic" displayed in the work of artists like Del Rey and Gomez, combined with the multiple celebrities speaking out about their mental health issues, reveals a complex media ecology. A star like Gomez can announce that she wants to empower women to feel allowed to fail while simultaneously creating art that flirts with romantic notions of suicide and psychic suffering.

On the one hand, Gomez speaking out about her issues and encouraging people to seek help can be considered as part of the postfeminist confidence trope. Encouraging women to "feel allowed to fall apart" can be another way of "empowering" them to take responsibility for their own lives. Even more so if the help one is encouraged to seek is to turn to the traditional psychiatric system, following the victim-to-victor narrative and understanding one's sadness as caused entirely by neurological components. This approach does require a reaching out for help, but not in a messy, (directly) interpersonal way. The trust in the psychiatric system maintains mental illness as something singular to be taken care of just as a "traditional" physical disease. If the subject takes care of her issues through medical channels, she can remain a "no-needs woman" in all other areas of her life.

On the other hand, the increased presence of sadness and the raised awareness of mental illness as something that affects a lot of people can be seen as an acknowledgment of the impossibility of constant confidence and independence. Are Lovato, Gomez, Del Rey, and others signs that the self-disciplining of emotions, the need to be independent and strong is disappearing or loosening up? Is the makeup of the postfeminist and neoliberal subject changing so as to include (certain kinds of) vulnerability?

What is clear is that female celebrities suffering emotionally and sharing that with fans is not as much of a tarnish on their personal brands as such revelations once were. Instead an openness about mental health struggles can add to the authenticity of a celebrity brand, especially if the star herself is shown as working diligently to become better. In the case of Lovato and Gomez, the fact that they keep encountering obstacles and subsequently go into treatment, only makes them more authentic and relatable to their fans. The popularity of del Rey's persona and her sad music influenced and paved the way for the more straightforward sadness of a later artist like Billie Eilish.

Employing the lens of Orgad and Gill's confidence culture, the expression of vulnerability seen in these media narratives primarily serves to make the confident woman relatable and add authenticity.[164] And in McRobbie's understanding of the perfect-imperfect-resilience triad, the imperfect is only a limited expression of the constraints of the perfect, that always leads to a resilient bounce-back to perfection.[165] This does apply to Lovato and Gomez in the sense that their stories of weakness ultimately feed back into their celebrity brands as strong, independent women* and artists. But when it comes to del Rey, I would argue that it is a bit more complicated.

Opening up the artistic exploration of themes of dependency and vulnerability provides a space, however narrow, for sitting with the negative feelings instead of immediately trying to get rid of them. This aspect of sadness' emergence in the mainstream pop cultural landscape is further explored in the next chapter, where I examine how social media sad girls provide more spacious ways of feeling bad.

Conclusion

Celebrities are an important part of the pop cultural landscape and the ways they approach mental health function as models for how to think about such issues in culture at large. The shift from media speculation about what ailments a celebrity might suffer from (often in sensationalist ways) to a climate where stars themselves speak firsthand about their experiences indicates a turn toward more mental health-aware, intimate, and relatable celebrity branding strategies.

The case of Demi Lovato shows how celebrity health narratives around mental illness have changed throughout the 2010s. Their first tell-all documentary from 2012 was focused largely on presenting a star who had overcome difficulties and emerged stronger on the other side (down to the title of the film being *Stay Strong*). Even if Lovato showed some vulnerability, the focus was on how they had emerged from past difficulties, resembling the victim-to-victor narrative in which a diagnosis is made, treatment is had, and the subject is declared a winner over the disease. Their second tell-all documentary, released five years later, presents a more complicated picture of mental illness and recovery (and aptly titled *Simply Complicated*). The original illness narrative is questioned in the confession about Lovato being under the influence while filming the first documentary, and the viewer is subsequently presented with an individual who is flawed and constantly working on their issues, which appear as always in need of management. This suggests that the ideal neoliberal and postfeminist subject now has room for some failure and weakness, but these have to be worked at to be repeatedly overcome. Lovato's 2018 relapse, the profitable release of the single Sober, and the subsequent comeback in 2020 cement Lovato's narrative as one of successful self-transformation and reinvention. This was only heightened with the third tell-all documentary series about the singer's overdose that was released in 2021 (where Lovato's struggles with their inner demons were hinted at in the title *Dancing with the devil*). While the celebrities who managed to go through public breakdowns and come out stronger on the other side in previous eras tended to be male, Lovato's narrative suggests that this is no longer the case and that female* stars can now also recast themselves as successful masters of their own lives by overcoming difficulties. The gendered aspect of the celebrity mental illness narrative is now not configured so as to invalidate female celebrities who suffer, instead the female star who is depressed or anxious and successfully manages it fits well into the dominant "psychic life" of neoliberalism, postfeminism, and a market-friendly popular feminism. The fact that Lovato has since defined their gender identity as non-binary does not take away from the gendered meaning of their celebrity health narrative. Instead it shows that sharing experiences of traumatic events and having them strengthen one's authenticity is available to celebrities across the gender spectrum.

The female illness narrative is emphasized in the case of Selena Gomez, who at the start of the decade was defined as a "super can-do girl" who stayed far away from scandal,[166] but then opened up about her experience of depression and anxiety in 2016. She has largely been cast as a mental health advocate and responsible role model, and her case shows the viability/marketability of mental health advocacy for a celebrity brand at that point in time. This has been further highlighted in Gomez's makeup line, *Rare*, which is marketed as a mental health aware brand where 1 % of sales go to support mental health.[167] The line even includes the "Stay Vulnerable Liquid Eyeshadow" which Gomez herself describes as celebrating "the soft, flushed look we get when we feel the most vulnerable."[168] In this instance it is quite literally vulnerability that is being sold, down to the description of how one might look after a day of crying.

At the same time, Gomez has played with a sad aesthetic in her work as an artist and television producer. Comparing how her work was received with Lana del Rey's debut in 2011-2012 revealed the shifting attitudes toward expressions of female sadness and weakness. The subsequent success of del Rey and the broader turn in popular culture toward more sad expressions suggest a dissatisfaction with overtly positive empowerment narratives and a yearning by audiences for representations of negative affects like sadness. Something I discuss further in the following chapter, which looks at the worlds of social media and how mental illness and sadness have been discussed there.

Lovato and Gomez are examples of profitable vulnerability, while del Rey is more aligned with the sad girl culture I discuss in the following chapter, since her expression of sadness is not something already overcome in the past but is being explored as it is experienced.

NOTES

1. Beck et al, *Celebrity Health Narratives and the Public Health.*
2. McNamara, "Lady Gaga Penned a Letter About Living With PTSD."
3. Franssen, "The celebritization of self-care," 91; see also Bell, "From bad girl to mad girl;" Fisher, "We Love This Trainwreck!;" Harper, *Madness, Power and the Media*; Holmes, "Little Lena's a Big Girl Now."
4. In May 2021 Demi Lovato came out as non-binary and announced that they will use the pronouns they/them, Blistein, "Demi Lovato Comes Out as Gender Non-Binary." Despite this, I have kept Lovato as an example of how female celebrities mediate their mental health because the singer was a key figure in popular girl culture for the majority of their career up until this announcement. I am using the pronouns they/them to refer to Lovato in the text, but I have not changed the pronouns in older quotes referring to the star as she/her. I hope this slippage will not disturb the reader, but instead serve as a reminder of the fluidity of the gender spectrum.
5. I have culled these primarily from compilation articles such as Roberts, "39 Celebrities Who Have Opened Up About Mental Health," and van Eijk, "19 Celebrities Who Have Spoken Out About Their Anxiety." See also Altshul, "14 Celebrities Who Have Experienced Depression;" Bain, "What 17 Celebrities Have Said About Having Depression;" Felson, "Celebrities With Anxiety;" Forstadt, "Stars Who Have Opened Up About Dealing With Anxiety;" Gavilanes, "How Busy Philipps, Kendall Jenner & More Stars Who Battle Anxiety Deal with It;" Grant and Gomez, "14 Celebrities with Depression Get Real About Self-Care and Mental Health;" Hugel, "8 Celebrities Talk About Anxiety;" Naftulin, "15 Inspiring Things Celebrities Have Said About Dealing With Anxiety;" Nelson, "13 Celebrities With Anxiety Disorders;" Proudfoot, "Celebrities Speak Out About Their Mental Health Battles;" Ratini, "19 Celebrities With Depression;" Selzer, "Celebrities who have talked about anxiety;" Singh, "28 celebrities who have opened up about their struggles with mental illness;" Tannenbaum, "30 Celebrities Who Have Opened Up About Depression;" Truschel, "10 Actors Open Up About Their Battle with Depression;" Yagoda, "Gretchen Rossi, Chrissy Teigen & More Stars Who've Opened Up About Their Struggles with Postpartum Depression;" and Yagoda, "'It's Okay Not to Be Strong Sometimes.'" These listicles appeared on the sites of magazines like *Elle, Marie Claire, Seventeen, Harper's Bazaar*, the *Hollywood Reporter*, and *Good Housekeeping* as well as web-only publications like *Refinery29, Bustle, Buzzfeed*, and *Insider*. An additional few were also found on health-specific sites like WebMD, EverydayHealth.com, Psycom, and Health.com.

6. Abad-Santos, "Meghan Markle's honesty about suicidal thoughts in her Oprah interview could help others;" Emmanuele, "Paris Hilton Felt "Empowered" By Sharing Her Story of Past Abuse;" Osaka, "Naomi Osaka: 'It's O.K. Not to Be O.K.'"

7. 33 celebrities (31%) said they struggled with anxiety; 28 stars (27%) said they have experienced depression; 12 (11%) talked about having both depression and anxiety; 10 (10%) named postpartum depression; and 7 (7%) mentioned bipolar disorder.

8. Multiple of the stars have spoken about their issues several times, but I have only counted them once, and the numbers per year refer to when they talked about it the first time. I made this decision based on the assumption that the first time someone spoke out indicates what the perceptions around mental health and illness looked like in popular culture at the time.

9. Holmes and Negra, *In the Limelight and Under the Microscope*, 5.

10. Ibid, 5.

11. Luckett, "Toxic: The Implosion of Britney Spears's Star Image."

12. Melas, "Britney Spears' 13 year conservatorship has finally ended."

13. Duke, "Lindsay Lohan's troubled timeline."

14. Polaschek, "The dissonant personas of a female celebrity."

15. Koman, "Good News: Amanda Bynes Is Doing 'Really Well;'" Ruiz, "Amanda Bynes: A Reminder That Mental Health Woes Flourish in Our 20's?"

16. See "Got-You-Where-I-Want-You," Tumblr post, accessed June 22, 2022, http://got-you-where-i-want-you.tumblr.com/post/158824899040; "Sweet-Despondency," Tumblr post, accessed June 22, 2022, https://sweet-despondency.tumblr.com/post/147347687983/mothurs-candid-photo-of-lucifer-and-the-angel.

17. Cagle, "Mariah Carey: My Battle with Bipolar Disorder."

18. Marwick and boyd, "To see and be seen," 150.

19. Ingrassia, "My Nine-Year Struggle with Anorexia by Brittany Snow."

20. Truong, "Brittany Snow Spoke "Too Early" About Mental Health."

21. Ibid.

22. Newberry, "Britney Spears hasn't fully controlled her life for years."

23. Farrow and Tolentino, "Britney Spears's Conservatorship Nightmare."

24. Melas, "Britney Spears' 13 year conservatorship has finally ended;" Newberry, "Britney Spears hasn't fully controlled her life for years."

25. Steptoe, *Genius and the Mind*.

26. Harper, *Madness, Power and the Media*.

27. Franssen, "The celebritization of self-care," 95.

28. Nunn and Biressi, "'A trust betrayed': Celebrity and the work of emotion," 53.

29. Lerner, *When Illness Goes Public*, 8.
30. Harper, "Madly famous: Narratives of mental illness in celebrity culture," 314.
31. Martin, "'Does this film make me look fat?' Celebrity, gender and I'm still here," 31.
32. Ibid, 31.
33. Franssen, "The celebritization of self-care," 95; see also Bell, "The Insanity Plea;" Holmes, "Little Lena's a Big Girl Now," McLean, "Feeling and the Filmed Body."
34. Franssen, "The celebritization of self-care," 96.
35. Petersen, "How The 2010s Killed The Celebrity Gossip Machine."
36. Ibid.
37. Marwick and boyd, "To see and be seen," 139.
38. Ibid, 140, italicization in original.
39. Ibid, 139.
40. Nunn and Biressi, "'A trust betrayed': Celebrity and the work of emotion," 54.
41. Barker, Gill and Harvey, *Mediated intimacy*, 24, italicization in original.
42. Hearn and Schoenhoff, "From Celebrity to Influencer," 197-198.
43. Ibid, 200.
44. Ibid, 200.
45. Ibid, 200.
46. Khamis, Ang, and Welling, "Self-branding, 'micro-celebrity' and the rise of Social Media Influencers."
47. Orgad and Gill (2022) discuss the inverse of this, in the sense that some vulnerability is shared by confident women so as to make them relatable (p. 71).
48. Nunn and Biressi, "'A trust betrayed': Celebrity and the work of emotion," 49.
49. DeMoss, "Vloggers Changing the Dialogue on Mental Health;" Fergusson, "11 YouTubers Who Have Spoken Out About Their Struggles With Social Anxiety;" Tonic, "15 Beauty Vloggers Who Are Open About Mental Illness."
50. Berryman and Kavka, "'I Guess A Lot of People See Me as a Big Sister or a Friend,'" 85.
51. Ibid, 87.
52. Gamson, "The Unwatched Life Is Not Worth Living."
53. Ibid, 1065-1067.
54. Khamis, Ang, and Welling, "Self-branding, 'micro-celebrity' and the rise of Social Media Influencers."
55. Projansky, *Spectacular Girls*, 73-75; Ryals, *Best Friends Forever*; Rutherford, *Demi Lovato & Selena Gomez*; Willen, "Selena Gomez and Demi Lovato's friendship timeline."

56. Harris, *Future Girl.*
57. Ibid, 27.
58. Projansky, *Spectacular Girls*, 4.
59. Ibid, 4.
60. Ibid, 75, 93. Projansky also discusses the racialized aspect of Gomez's celebrity at length, arguing that her Mexican-American identity is downplayed in most media coverage, but her visibility still "potentially opens up reflection on mixed identities and provides a potential point of identification for mixed audiences."
61. Stables, "With Rare Beauty, Selena Gomez Has Rewritten the Script for Start-Ups."
62. Even though Lovato now identifies as non-binary, they were still an integral part of popular girl culture during the first part of their career.
63. Orgad and Gill, *Confidence Culture*, 96.
64. Ibid, 96.
65. McRobbie, *Feminism and the politics of resilience.*
66. Ibid, 43.
67. Bonner, "Inside Demi Lovato's Huge Net Worth."
68. Hunter, "Demi Lovato Rehab."
69. Cotliar, "Demi Lovato Has Bipolar Disorder."
70. Bell, "The Insanity Plea;" Holmes, "Little Lena's a Big Girl Now."
71. Franssen, "The celebritization of self-care," 96.
72. Russo (director), "Demi Lovato: Stay Strong."
73. Ibid, 96.
74. Gill and Orgad, "The Confidence Cult(ure)," Orgad and Gill, *Confidence Culture.*
75. Orgad and Gill, *Confidence Culture.*
76. Bell, "The Insanity Plea."
77. Ibid, 199.
78. Ibid, 201.
79. Ibid, 221.
80. Harris, *Future Girl.*
81. Franssen, "The celebritization of self-care," 98, italicization in original.
82. HuffPost, "The Lovato Treatment Scholarship;" Lovato, *Staying Strong: 365 Days a Year;* Lovato, *Staying Strong: A Journal;* Macrae, "Demi Lovato's Book Cracks The New York Times Best Seller List;"
83. Stutz, "Demi Lovato Releases Bipolar PSA, Announces Mental Health Listening & Engagement Tour."
84. CBS News, "Demi Lovato now co-owns rehab center where she received treatment;" Chan, "DNC 2016;" Puckett, "Demi Lovato Hosts Seminars With Fans Before Future Now Tour to Discuss Mental Health Issues."

85. Demi Lovato, "Demi Lovato: Simply Complicated—Official Documentary," Youtube video, October 17, 2017, accessed June 25, 2022, https://www.youtube.com/watch?v=ZWTlL_w8cRA.
86. Marwick and boyd, "To see and be seen."
87. Du Gay, *Consumption and identity at work*; Gill, "Postfeminist media culture;" Ringrose and Walkerdine, "Regulating The Abject."
88. Gill, "The affective, cultural and psychic life of postfeminism;" Scharff, "The Psychic Life of Neoliberalism."
89. Franssen, "The celebritization of self-care," 96.
90. Ibid, 96.
91. Martin, *Bipolar Expeditions.*
92. Franssen, "The celebritization of self-care," 92.
93. Illouz, *Cold Intimacies,* 55.
94. Ibid, 55.
95. Franssen, "The celebritization of self-care," 96.
96. Banet-Weiser, *Empowered*, 13.
97. Ibid, 13.
98. Orgad and Gill, *Confidence Culture.*
99. Blackman, "Psychiatric culture and bodies of resistance."
100. Franssen, "The celebritization of self-care," 99.
101. Gill, "Postfeminist media culture;" Gill "Culture and Subjectivity in Neoliberal and Postfeminist Times;" McRobbie, *The Aftermath of Feminism*; Ringrose and Walkerdine, "Regulating The Abject;" Scharff, "Gender and neoliberalism;"
102. Orgad and Gill, *Confidence Culture.*
103. Demi Lovato (ddlovato), "My truth... http://demilovato.co/sober #sober out now," Twitter, June 21, 2018, accessed June 25, 2022, https://twitter.com/ddlovato/status/1009807182089445377.
104. Romano, "Demi Lovato's Sober song reveals singer relapsed after six years."
105. RadarStaff, "Demi Lovato at War With Her Rehab Center Amid Relapse Confession."
106. Wang, "Demi Lovato Hospitalized for Apparent Drug Overdose."
107. Bailey, "Demi Lovato Makes First Statement After Hospitalization."
108. Recording Industry Association of America, Gold and Platinum Demi Lovato Sober, website, accessed June 25, 2022, https://www.riaa.com/gold-platinum/?tab_active=default-award&ar=DEMI+LOVATO&ti=SOBER.
109. Demi Lovato News (@demetriaaalove), "Lovatics I'm starting the hashtag #HowDemiHasHelpedMe. Please share your stories and positive things so hopefully Demi sees positive things if she comes online," Twitter, July 25, 2018, accessed June 25, 2022, https://twitter.com/demetriaaalove/status/1021964896819396610.

110. Amatulli, "Demi Lovato Fans Are Sharing Stories Of How She Helped Them;" Newsbeat, "Demi Lovato: 'How Demi has helped me' stories shared by fans;" Schuster, "How Fans Are Showing Demi Lovato She Can Still Be a Role Model After Her Relapse."
111. Harmonizer (@Enchanted5H), "#HowDemiHasHelpedMe P2: The Night I Attempted Suicide Demi Had a Performance on Tv. My Dad Was Watching It and Not Me. I Was Upstairs in My Room Taking Pills to," Twitter, July 25, 2018, accessed June 22, 2022, https://twitter.com/Enchanted5H/status/1021976397097709568.
112. Ibid.
113. Blackmon, "Demi Lovato Fans Staged A Tribute Concert For The Singer Days After She Was Hospitalized."
114. Kornhaber, "Demi Lovato Makes a Powerful Confession at the Grammys."
115. Demi Lovato, "Demi Lovato: Dancing With the Devil, YouTube Series, accessed June 22, 2022, https://www.youtube.com/playlist?list=PLy4Kg0J0TkearxiMrCsHih5xJzttUe8JC.
116. Spanos, "'Demi Lovato: Dancing With the Devil.'"
117. Demi Lovato, "Dancing With The Devil (Official Video)," Youtube video, accessed June 22, 2022, https://www.youtube.com/watch?v=EAg69LaLlS0.
118. Martins, "Billboard Cover: Selena Gomez on Her New Chapter."
119. Caulfield, "Selena Gomez Earns Third No. 1 Album on Billboard 200 Chart With 'Rare.'"
120. Bonner, "What Is Selena Gomez's Net Worth and 'Only Murders' Salary?"
121. Bailey, "Selena Gomez and Justin Bieber Drama Timeline;" Wallace, "A complete history of Justin Bieber and Selena Gomez's relationship."
122. Martins, "Billboard Cover: Selena Gomez on Her New Chapter."
123. Chiu, "Selena Gomez Taking Time Off After Dealing with 'Anxiety, Panic Attacks and Depression' Due to Her Lupus Diagnosis."
124. Ibid.
125. Mei, "Watch Selena Gomez's Empowering, Emotional Acceptance Speech at the AMAs."
126. Avila, "Selena Gomez's AMAs Acceptance Speech Was a Heartfelt One;" Rosa, "Selena Gomez Tears Up During Her Emotional Speech at the American Music Awards 2016;" Vogue.com, "Selena Gomez Breaks Her Silence at the AMAs."
127. Vogue.com, "Selena Gomez Gets Real About Anxiety—And How Therapy Changed Everything."
128. Brown, "Selena Gomez Is Grown Up, in Love, and Taking Control of Her Mental Health."

129. Willis and Drysdale, "Selena Gomez Hospitalized For Mental Health."
130. Langford, "Selena Gomez's Wild Ride."
131. Wang, "Selena Gomez Is Taking a Social Media Break;" Willis and Drysdale, "Selena Gomez Hospitalized For Mental Health."
132. Bonner, "Selena Gomez Reportedly in Mental Health Facility After Being Hospitalized for 'Emotional Breakdown.'"
133. Franssen, "The celebritization of self-care," 95.
134. Dodson, "Selena Gomez Broke Her Instagram Silence to Reflect on 2018."
135. Longman, "Selena Gomez Shares Brutal Reality of her 2019 Treatment."
136. Vivinetto, "Selena Gomez reveals bipolar disorder diagnosis."
137. Incidentally, this was the same hospital that Sylvia Plath stayed at in the 1950s and later chronicled in *The Bell Jar*. Other famous former patients include poet Anne Sexton and singer Marianne Faithfull; Conradt, "10 Famous Residents of McLean Psychiatric Hospital."
138. Vivinetto, "Selena Gomez reveals bipolar disorder diagnosis."
139. Bailey, "Selena Gomez Reveals to Miley Cyrus That She Was Diagnosed With Bipolar Disorder;" CBBCNewsround, "Selena Gomez: Singer speaks about bipolar disorder;" Scott, "Selena Gomez reveals bipolar disorder diagnosis;" Vivinetto, "Selena Gomez reveals bipolar disorder diagnosis;" Young, "Selena Gomez opens up about bipolar diagnosis for first time during Instagram Live with Miley Cyrus."
140. Luu, "Selena Gomez Explained Why She Revealed Her Bipolar Disorder Diagnosis On Miley Cyrus's Show."
141. Saint Louis, "For Families of Teens at Suicide Risk, '13 Reasons' Raises Concerns."
142. Alderton, *The aesthetics of self-harm.*
143. Carlin, "The Powerful Meaning Behind Selena Gomez's Bracelet In Her 'Bad Liar' Photo."
144. Plaugic, "Selena Gomez releases new vertical music video you can only watch on Spotify's mobile app."
145. Alderton, *The aesthetics of self-harm.*
146. Heaf, "Woman Of The Year: Lana Del Rey."
147. Cassan, "Lana Del Rey:'Je me sens l'âme d'une guerrière;'" Wagner, "Billboard Cover: Lana Del Rey on Why Her Pop Stardom 'Could Easily Not Have Happened.'"
148. Jonze, "Lana Del Rey: 'I wish I was dead already.'"
149. Schrodt, "Lana Del Rey's Feminist Problem;" Vigier, "The Meaning of Lana Del Rey."
150. Shugerman, "Lana Del Rey: Not A Feminist."
151. Vogue.com, "Selena Gomez Gets Real About Anxiety—And How Therapy Changed Everything."

152. Vigier, "The Meaning of Lana Del Rey," 3, 1.
153. Alderton, *The aesthetics of self-harm*, 100.
154. Ibid, 100.
155. Vogue.com, "Selena Gomez Gets Real About Anxiety—And How Therapy Changed Everything."
156. Banet-Weiser, *Empowered*, 13.
157. Horner, "This is how Lana Del Rey kickstarted a sad-pop revolution."
158. Interiano et al, "Musical trends and predictability of success in contemporary songs in and out of the top charts."
159. Ibid, 1.
160. Messman, "2020 Grammy Winners;" Nicholson, "Billie Eilish: the candid, self-aware voice of a generation takes on 007."
161. Horner, "This is how Lana Del Rey kickstarted a sad-pop revolution."
162. Ibid.
163. Ibid.
164. Orgad and Gill, *Confidence Culture*.
165. McRobbie, *Feminism and the politics of resilience*.
166. Projansky, *Spectacular Girls*, 75.
167. Stables, "With Rare Beauty, Selena Gomez Has Rewritten the Script for Start-Ups."
168. Rare Beauty, "Stay Vulnerable Liquid Eyeshadow," website, accessed June 25, 2022, https://www.rarebeauty.com/products/stay-vulnerable-liquid-eyeshadow?variant=34777545212039.

References

Abad-Santos, Alex. "Meghan Markle's Honesty about Suicidal Thoughts in Her Oprah Interview Could Help Others." *Vox*, March 8, 2021. https://www.vox.com/22320404/meghan-markle-suicide-oprah-cbs-interview.
Alderton, Zoe. *The Aesthetics of Self-Harm: The Visual Rhetoric of Online Self-Harm Communities*. London and New York: Routledge, 2018. https://doi.org/10.4324/9781315637853-2.
Altshul, Sara. "14 Celebrities Who Have Experienced Depression." *EverydayHealth. Com*, March 4, 2016. https://www.everydayhealth.com/pictures/celebrities-who-have-experienced-depression/.
Amatulli, Jenna. "Demi Lovato Fans Are Sharing Stories Of How She Helped Them." *HuffPost*, July 25, 2018. https://www.huffpost.com/entry/demi-lovato-fans-are-sharing-their-stories-about-how-she-helped-them_n_5b587dd9e4b0fd5c73caa772.
Avila, Theresa. "Selena Gomez's AMAs Acceptance Speech Was a Heartfelt One." *TheCut.Com*, November 21, 2016. https://www.thecut.com/2016/11/selena-gomez-amas-acceptance-speech-was-a-heartfelt-one.html.

Bailey, Alyssa. "Demi Lovato Makes First Statement After Hospitalization: 'I Will Keep Fighting.'" *Elle.Com*, August 5, 2018. https://www.elle.com/culture/celebrities/a22647049/demi-lovato-first-statement-after-overdose-hospitalization/.

Bailey, Alyssa. "Selena Gomez and Justin Bieber Drama Timeline—Jelena Breakup Drama Timeline." *Elle.Com*, October 23, 2019. https://www.elle.com/culture/celebrities/news/a38542/justin-bieber-selena-gomez-relationship-drama-timeline/.

Bailey, Alyssa. "Selena Gomez Reveals To Miley Cyrus That She Was Diagnosed With Bipolar Disorder." *Elle.Com*, April 3, 2020. https://www.elle.com/culture/celebrities/a32036287/selena-gomez-miley-cyrus-bipolar-interview/.

Bain, Lisa. "What 17 Celebrities Have Said About Having Depression, In Their Own Words." *Goodhousekeeping.Com*, June 19, 2019. https://www.goodhousekeeping.com/health/wellness/g3541/celebrities-with-depression/.

Banet-Weiser, Sarah. *Empowered: Popular Feminism and Popular Misogyny*. Durham and London: Duke University Press, 2018.

Barker, Meg-John, Rosalind Gill, and Laura Harvey. *Mediated Intimacy: Sex Advice in Media Culture*. Cambridge: Polity, 2018.

Beck, Christina S., Stellina M.A. Chapman, Nathaniel Simmons, Kelly E. Tenzek, and Stephanie M. Ruhl. *Celebrity Health Narratives and the Public Health*. Jefferson, NC: McFarland & Company, 2015.

Bell, Emma. "From Bad Girl to Mad Girl: British Female Celebrity, Reality Products, and the Pathologization of Pop-Feminism." *Genders* 48 (2008).

Bell, Emma. "The Insanity Plea: Female Celebrities, Reality Media and the Psychopathology of British Pop-Feminism." In *In the Limelight and Under the Microscope: Forms and Functions of Female Celebrity*, edited by Diane Negra and Su Holmes, 199–223. New York & London: Continuum Books, 2011.

Berryman, Rachel, and Misha Kavka. "'I Guess A Lot of People See Me as a Big Sister or a Friend': The Role of Intimacy in the Celebrification of Beauty Vloggers." *Journal of Gender Studies* 26, no. 3 (2017): 307–20. https://doi.org/10.1080/09589236.2017.1288611.

Blackman, Lisa. "Psychiatric Culture and Bodies of Resistance." *Body & Society* 13, no. 2 (2007): 1–23. https://doi.org/10.1177/1357034X07077770.

Blackmon, Michael. "Demi Lovato Fans Staged A Tribute Concert For The Singer Days After She Was Hospitalized." *Buzzfeed News*, July 27, 2018. https://www.buzzfeednews.com/article/michaelblackmon/demi-fans.

Blistein, Jon. "Demi Lovato Comes Out as Gender Non-Binary." *Rolling Stone*, May 19, 2021. https://www.rollingstone.com/music/music-news/demi-lovato-non-binary-coming-out-pronouns-1171379/.

Bonner, Mehera. "Selena Gomez Reportedly in Mental Health Facility After Being Hospitalized for 'Emotional Breakdown.'" *Cosmopolitan.Com*, October 11,

2018. https://www.cosmopolitan.com/entertainment/a23714201/selena-gomez-reportedly-in-mental-health-facility-after-being-hospitalized-for-emotional-breakdown/.

Bonner, Mehera. "Inside Demi Lovato's Huge Net Worth: Music, Disney, and Touring." *Cosmopolitan*, January 20, 2022a. https://www.cosmopolitan.com/entertainment/celebs/a38829448/demi-lovato-net-worth/.

Bonner, Mehera. "What Is Selena Gomez's Net Worth and 'Only Murders' Salary?" *Cosmopolitan*, March 21, 2022b. https://www.cosmopolitan.com/entertainment/celebs/a39489561/selena-gomez-net-worth/.

Brown, Laura. "Selena Gomez Is Grown Up, in Love, and Taking Control of Her Mental Health." *InStyle*, August 3, 2017. https://www.instyle.com/celebrity/selena-gomez-cover-story.

Cagle, Jess. "Mariah Carey: My Battle with Bipolar Disorder." *People.Com*, April 11, 2018. https://people.com/music/mariah-carey-bipolar-disorder-diagnosis-exclusive/.

Carlin, Shannon. "The Powerful Meaning Behind Selena Gomez's Bracelet In Her 'Bad Liar' Photo." *Refinery29*, May 17, 2017. http://www.refinery29.com/2017/05/154913/selena-gomez-bad-liar-bracelet-meaning.

Cassan, Félicien. "Lana Del Rey:"Je Me Sens l'âme d'une Guerrière"." *Madame Figaro*, June 27, 2014. http://madame.lefigaro.fr/celebrites/lana-del-rey-sens-lame-dune-guerriere-270614-875074.

Caulfield, Keith. "Selena Gomez Earns Third No. 1 Album on Billboard 200 Chart With 'Rare.'" *Billboard.Com*, January 21, 2020. https://www.billboard.com/articles/business/chart-beat/8548614/selena-gomez-rare-number-one-billboard-200-albums-chart.

CBBCNewsround. "Selena Gomez: Singer Speaks about Bipolar Disorder." *BBC.Co.Uk*, April 6, 2020. https://www.bbc.co.uk/newsround/52174172.

CBSNews. "Demi Lovato Now Co-Owns Rehab Center Where She Received Treatment." *CBSNews.Com*, September 8, 2016. https://www.cbsnews.com/news/demi-lovato-now-co-owns-rehab-center-where-she-received-treatment/.

Chan, Amanda. "DNC 2016: Demi Lovato Urges Politicians to Support Laws Improving Health Care Access." *Teen Vogue*, July 26, 2016. https://www.teenvogue.com/story/demi-lovato-dnc-2016-mental-health-care-acess-laws.

Chiu, Melody. "Selena Gomez Taking Time Off After Dealing with 'Anxiety, Panic Attacks and Depression' Due to Her Lupus Diagnosis." *People.Com*, August 30, 2016. https://people.com/celebrity/selena-gomez-taking-a-break-after-lupus-complications/.

Conradt, Stacy. "10 Famous Residents of McLean Psychiatric Hospital." *Mental Floss*, February 13, 2013. https://www.mentalfloss.com/article/48872/10-famous-residents-mclean-psychiatric-hospital.

Cotliar, Sharon. "Demi Lovato Has Bipolar Disorder." *People.Com*, April 20, 2011. https://people.com/celebrity/demi-lovato-has-bipolar-disorder/.

DeMoss, Dustin. "Vloggers Changing the Dialogue on Mental Health." *Huffingtonpost*, April 13, 2015. http://www.huffingtonpost.com/dustin-demoss/vloggers-changing-the-dia_b_6650914.html.

Dodson, Claire P. "Selena Gomez Broke Her Instagram Silence to Reflect on 2018." *Teen Vogue*, January 14, 2019. https://www.teenvogue.com/story/selena-gomez-broke-instagram-silence-reflect-2018.

Gay, Paul Du. *Consumption and Identity at Work*. London, Thousand Oaks, New Dehli: SAGE Publications, 1996.

Duke, Alan. "Lindsay Lohan's Troubled Timeline." *CNN.Com*, March 29, 2012. https://edition.cnn.com/2012/03/28/showbiz/lohan-troubled-timeline/index.html.

Emmanuele, Julia. "Paris Hilton Felt 'Empowered' By Sharing Her Story Of Past Abuse." *Bustle.Com*, September 12, 2020. https://www.bustle.com/entertainment/paris-hilton-felt-empowered-by-sharing-story-of-past-abuse.

Farrow, Ronan, and Jia Tolentino. "Britney Spears's Conservatorship Nightmare." *The New Yorker*, July 3, 2021. https://www.newyorker.com/news/american-chronicles/britney-spears-conservatorship-nightmare.

Felson, Sabrina. "Celebrities With Anxiety." *WebMD.Com*, July 21, 2018. https://www.webmd.com/anxiety-panic/ss/slideshow-celebrities-anxiety.

Fergusson, Caroline. "11 YouTubers Who Have Spoken Out About Their Struggles With Social Anxiety." *MTV UK*, April 26, 2017. http://www.mtv.co.uk/life/news/11-youtubers-who-have-spoken-out-about-their-struggles-with-social-anxiety.

Fisher, Anna Watkins. "We Love This Trainwreck! Sacrificing Britney to Save America." In *In the Limelight and Under the Microscope*, edited by Su Holmes and Diane Negra, 303–32. New York & London: Continuum Books, 2011. https://doi.org/10.5040/9781628928082.ch-014.

Forstadt, Jillian. "Stars Who Have Opened Up About Dealing With Anxiety." *Hollywoodreporter.Com*, July 19, 2018. https://www.hollywoodreporter.com/lists/celebs-anxiety-ryan-reynolds-lena-dunham-more-mental-health-1124846.

Franssen, Gaston. "The Celebritization of Self-Care: The Celebrity Health Narrative of Demi Lovato and the Sickscape of Mental Illness." *European Journal of Cultural Studies* 23, no. 1 (2020): 89–111. https://doi.org/10.1177/1367549419861636.

Gamson, Joshua. "The Unwatched Life Is Not Worth Living: The Elevation of the Ordinary in Celebrity Culture." *PMLA* 126, no. 4 (2011): 1061–69.

Gavilanes, Grace. "How Busy Philipps, Kendall Jenner & More Stars Who Battle Anxiety Deal with It." *People.Com*, May 31, 2018. https://people.com/health/celebs-overcome-anxiety/.

Gill, Rosalind. "Postfeminist Media Culture: Elements of a Sensibility." *European Journal of Cultural Studies* 10, no. 2 (May 1, 2007): 147–66. https://doi.org/10.1177/1367549407075898.

Gill, Rosalind. "Culture and Subjectivity in Neoliberal and Postfeminist Times." *Subjectivity* 25 (2008): 432–45. https://doi.org/10.1057/sub.2008.28.

Gill, Rosalind. "The Affective, Cultural and Psychic Life of Postfeminism: A Postfeminist Sensibility 10 Years On." *European Journal of Cultural Studies* 20, no. 6 (2017): 606–26. https://doi.org/10.1177/1367549417733003.

Gill, Rosalind, and Shani Orgad. "The Confidence Cult(Ure)." *Australian Feminist Studies* 30, no. 86 (2015): 324–44.

Grant, Stacey, and Jasmine Gomez. "14 Celebrities with Depression Get Real About Self-Care and Mental Health." *Seventeen.Com*, April 17, 2019. https://www.seventeen.com/celebrity/celebrity-couples/g24667606/famous-celebrities-with-depression/.

Harper, Stephen. "Madly Famous: Narratives of Mental Illness in Celebrity Culture." In *Framing Celebrity: New Directions in Celebrity Culture*, edited by Su Holmes and Sean Redmond, 311–27. London: Routledge, 2006.

Harper, Stephen. *Madness, Power and the Media: Class, Gender and Race in Popular Representations of Mental Distress*. Basingstoke: Palgrave Macmillan, 2009.

Harris, Anita. *Future Girl: Young Women in the Twenty-First Century*. New York & London: Routledge, 2004.

Heaf, Jonathan. "Woman Of The Year: Lana Del Rey." *GQ*, October 1, 2012. https://www.gq-magazine.co.uk/article/woman-of-the-year-lana-del-rey.

Hearn, Alison, and Stephanie Schoenhoff. "From Celebrity to Influencer: Tracing the Diffusion of Celebrity Value across the Data Stream." In *A Companion to Celebrity*, edited by P. David Marshall and Sean Redmond, 194–212. Malden, MA, Oxford, and West Sussex: John Wiley & Sons, Inc., 2016. https://doi.org/10.1002/9781118475089.ch11.

Holmes, Su. "Little Lena's a Big Girl Now." *Feminist Media Studies* 15, no. 5 (2015): 813–28. https://doi.org/10.1080/14680777.2014.995117.

Holmes, Su, and Diane Negra, eds. *In the Limelight and Under the Microscope: Forms and Functions of Female Celebrity*. New York & London: Continuum Books, 2011.

Horner, Al. "This Is How Lana Del Rey Kickstarted a Sad-Pop Revolution." *Redbull.Com*, August 30, 2019. https://www.redbull.com/se-en/lana-del-rey-sad-pop-revolution.

HuffPost. "The Lovato Treatment Scholarship: Demi Announces Program To Assist Those With Mental Illness." *Huffpost.Com*, June 27, 2013. https://www.huffpost.com/entry/the-lovato-treatment-scholarship-demi_n_3511726.

Hugel, Melissa. "8 Celebrities Talk About Anxiety—And Teach Us How to Deal With Ours." *Mic.Com*, September 22, 2015. https://www.mic.com/articles/125647/jennifer-lawrence-lena-dunham-and-chris-evans-live-with-anxiety-and-they-taught-us-how-to-deal-with-ours.

Hunter, Aina. "Demi Lovato Rehab: Why Is Disney Star Seeking Help?" *CBSNews.Com*, November 2, 2010. https://www.cbsnews.com/news/demi-lovato-rehab-why-is-disney-star-seeking-help/.

Illouz, Eva. *Cold Intimacies: The Making of Emotional Capitalism*. Cambridge, UK and Malden, MA: Polity Press, 2007.

Ingrassia, Lisa. "My Nine-Year Struggle with Anorexia by Brittany Snow." *People. Com*, October 15, 2007. https://people.com/archive/my-nine-year-struggle-with-anorexia-by-brittany-snow-vol-68-no-16/.

Interiano, Myra, Kamyar Kazemi, Lijia Wang, Jienian Yang, Zhaoxia Yu, and Natalia L. Komarova. "Musical Trends and Predictability of Success in Contemporary Songs in and out of the Top Charts." *Royal Society Open Science* 5, no. 5 (2018). https://doi.org/10.1098/rsos.171274.

Jonze, Tim. "Lana Del Rey: 'I Wish I Was Dead Already.'" *The Guardian*, June 12, 2014. https://www.theguardian.com/music/2014/jun/12/lana-del-rey-ultraviolence-album.

Khamis, Susie, Lawrence Ang, and Raymond Welling. "Self-Branding, 'Micro-Celebrity' and the Rise of Social Media Influencers." *Celebrity Studies* 8, no. 2 (2017): 191–208. https://doi.org/10.1080/19392397.2016.1218292.

Koman, Tess. "Good News: Amanda Bynes Is Doing 'Really Well.'" *Cosmopolitan. Com*, March 28, 2014. https://www.cosmopolitan.com/entertainment/celebs/news/a22765/amanda-bynes-doing-well/.

Kornhaber, Spencer. "Demi Lovato Makes a Powerful Confession at the Grammys." *The Atlantic*, January 27, 2020. https://www.theatlantic.com/culture/archive/2020/01/demi-lovatos-beautiful-shocking-grammys-song-anyone/605509/.

Langford, Katherine. "Selena Gomez's Wild Ride." Harper's Bazaar, February 7, 2018. https://www.harpersbazaar.com/culture/features/a15895669/selena-gomez-interview/.

Lerner, Barron H. *When Illness Goes Public: Celebrity Patients and How We Look at Medicine*. Baltimore, MD: John Hopkins University Press, 2006.

Longman, Molly. "Selena Gomez Shares Brutal Reality of Her 2019 Treatment." *Refinery29*, September 26, 2019. https://www.refinery29.com/en-us/2019/09/8485324/selena-gomez-opens-up-mental-health-award.

Lovato, Demi. *Staying Strong: 365 Days a Year*. New York: Feiwel and Friends, 2013.

Lovato, Demi. *Staying Strong: A Journal*. New York: Feiwel and Friends, 2014.

Luckett, Moya. "Toxic: The Implosion of Britney Spears's Star Image." *The Velvet Light Trap* 65, no. 1 (2010): 39–41. https://doi.org/10.1353/vlt.0.0077.

Luu, Christopher. "Selena Gomez Explained Why She Revealed Her Bipolar Disorder Diagnosis On Miley Cyrus's Show." *InStyle* , May 5, 2020. https://www.instyle.com/news/selena-gomez-bipolar-disorder-miley-cyrus-instagram-show.

Macrae, Dan. "Demi Lovato's Book Cracks The New York Times Best Seller List." *ETCanada.Com*, December 2, 2013. https://etcanada.com/news/90558/demi-lovatos-book-cracks-the-new-york-times-best-seller-list/.

Martin, Emily. *Bipolar Expeditions: Mania and Depression in American Culture.* Princeton University Press, 2009.

Martin, Nina K. "'Does This Film Make Me Look Fat?' Celebrity, Gender and I'm Still Here." In *Star Bodies and the Erotics of Suffering*, edited by Rebecca Bell-Metereau and Colleen Glenn, 29–54. Detroit, MI: Wayne State University Press, 2015.

Martins, Chris. "Billboard Cover: Selena Gomez on Her New Chapter—'I've Deserved This. I Earned It. This Is All Me.'" *Billboard.Com*, October 8, 2015. https://www.billboard.com/articles/news/cover-story/6721941/selena-gomez-revival-album-taylor-swift-justin-bieber-lupus-empowerment.

Marwick, Alice, and Danah Boyd. "To See and Be Seen: Celebrity Practice on Twitter." *Convergence* 17, no. 2 (2011): 139–58. https://doi.org/10.1177/1354856510394539.

McLean, Adrienne L. "Feeling and the Filmed Body: Judy Garland and the Kinesics of Suffering." *Film Quarterly* 55, no. 3 (2002): 2–15.

McRobbie, Angela. *The Aftermath of Feminism: Gender, Culture and Social Change.* London, Thousand Oaks, New Delhi and Singapore: SAGE, 2009.

McRobbie, Angela. *Feminism and the Politics of Resilience: Essays on Gender, Media and the End of Welfare.* Cambridge and Medford: Polity Press, 2020.

Mei, Gina. "Watch Selena Gomez's Empowering, Emotional Acceptance Speech at the AMAs." *Cosmopolitan*, November 21, 2016. https://www.cosmopolitan.com/entertainment/tv/a8346473/selena-gomez-acceptance-speech-amas-best-female-artist/.

Melas, Chloe. "Britney Spears' 13 Year Conservatorship Has Finally Ended." *CNN.Com*, November 12, 2021. https://edition.cnn.com/2021/11/12/entertainment/britney-spears-conservatorship-ends/index.html.

Messman, Lauren. "2020 Grammy Winners: Billie Eilish, Lizzo and All the Rest." *New York Times*, January 26, 2020. https://www.nytimes.com/2020/01/26/arts/music/grammy-winners.html.

Naftulin, Julia. "15 Inspiring Things Celebrities Have Said About Dealing With Anxiety." *Health.Com*, August 23, 2016. https://www.health.com/anxiety/celeb-struggle-anxiety.

Nelson, Calley. "13 Celebrities With Anxiety Disorders." *EverydayHealth.Com*, November 12, 2018. https://www.everydayhealth.com/anxiety-pictures/celebrities-with-anxiety-disorders.aspx.

Newberry, Laura. "Britney Spears Hasn't Fully Controlled Her Life for Years. Fans Insist It's Time to #FreeBritney." *Los Angeles Times*, September 18, 2019. https://www.latimes.com/california/story/2019-09-17/britney-spears-conservatorship-free-britney.

Newsbeat. "Demi Lovato: 'How Demi Has Helped Me' Stories Shared by Fans." *BBC.Com*, July 25, 2018. https://www.bbc.com/news/newsbeat-44952430.

Nicholson, Rebecca. "Billie Eilish: The Candid, Self-Aware Voice of a Generation Takes on 007." *The Guardian*, January 18, 2020. https://www.theguardian.com/music/2020/jan/18/billie-eilish-profile-bond-theme.

Nunn, Heather, and Anita Biressi. "'A Trust Betrayed': Celebrity and the Work of Emotion." *Celebrity Studies* 1, no. 1 (2010): 49–64. https://doi.org/10.1080/19392390903519065.

Orgad, Shani, and Rosalind Gill. *Confidence Culture.* Durham and London: Duke University Press, 2022. https://doi.org/10.1215/9781478021834.

Osaka, Naomi. "Naomi Osaka: 'It's O.K. Not to Be O.K.'" *TIME*, July 8, 2021. https://time.com/6077128/naomi-osaka-essay-tokyo-olympics/.

Petersen, Anne Helen. "How The 2010s Killed The Celebrity Gossip Machine." *BuzzFeed News*, December 26, 2019. https://www.buzzfeednews.com/article/annehelenpetersen/decade-celebrity-gossip-tabloids-paparazzi-social-media.

Plaugic, Lizzie. "Selena Gomez Releases New Vertical Music Video You Can Only Watch on Spotify's Mobile App." The Verge, May 18, 2017. https://www.theverge.com/2017/5/18/15658542/selena-gomez-music-video-bad-liar-watch-spotify.

Polaschek, Bronwyn. "The Dissonant Personas of a Female Celebrity: Amy and the Public Self of Amy Winehouse." *Celebrity Studies* 9, no. 1 (2018): 17–33. https://doi.org/10.1080/19392397.2017.1321490.

Projansky, Sarah. *Spectacular Girls: Media Fascination and Celebrity Culture.* New York & London: New York University Press, 2014.

Proudfoot, Jenny. "Celebrities Speak Out About Their Mental Health Battles." *Marieclaire.Co.Uk*, October 10, 2019. https://www.marieclaire.co.uk/news/celebrity-news/celebrities-speak-out-about-mental-health-12047.

Puckett, Lily. "Demi Lovato Hosts Seminars With Fans Before Future Now Tour to Discuss Mental Health Issues." *Teen Vogue*, July 13, 2016. https://www.teenvogue.com/story/demi-lovato-seminars-mental-health-substance-abuse-future-now-tour.

RadarStaff. "Demi Lovato at War With Her Rehab Center Amid Relapse Confession." *Radaronline.Com*, June 25, 2018. https://radaronline.com/videos/demi-lovato-at-war-with-rehab-center-amid-relapse-confession/.

Ratini, Melinda. "19 Celebrities With Depression." *WebMD.Com*, March 22, 2018. https://www.webmd.com/depression/ss/slideshow-depression-celebs.

Ringrose, Jessica, and Valerie Walkerdine. "Regulating The Abject: The TV Makeover as Site of Neo-Liberal Reinvention toward Bourgeois Femininity." *Feminist Media Studies* 8, no. 3 (2008): 227–46. https://doi.org/10.1080/14680770802217279.

Roberts, Kayleigh. "39 Celebrities Who Have Opened Up About Mental Health." *Harper's Bazaar*, January 14, 2018. https://www.harpersbazaar.com/celebrity/latest/g15159447/celebrities-depression-anxiety-mental-health/.

Romano, Nick. "Demi Lovato's Sober Song Reveals Singer Relapsed after Six Years." *EW.Com*, June 21, 2018. https://ew.com/music/2018/06/21/demi-lovato-sober-song-video/.

Rosa, Christopher. "Selena Gomez Tears Up During Her Emotional Speech at the American Music Awards 2016." *Glamour.Com*, November 21, 2016. https://www.glamour.com/story/selena-gomez-emotional-speech-american-music-awards-2016.

Ruiz, Michelle. "Amanda Bynes: A Reminder That Mental Health Woes Flourish in Our 20's?" *Cosmopolitan.Com*, May 28, 2013. https://www.cosmopolitan.com/entertainment/celebs/news/a13035/amanda-bynes-psychiatric-issues/.

Russo, Davi (director). *Demi Lovato: Stay Strong*. USA: MTV, 2012.

Rutherford, Lucy. *Demi Lovato & Selena Gomez: The Unofficial Story*. ECW Press, 2009.

Ryals, Lexi. *Best Friends Forever: Selena Gomez & Demi Lovato*. Price Stern Sloan, 2008.

Louis, Catherine Saint. "For Families of Teens at Suicide Risk, '13 Reasons' Raises Concerns." *New York Times*, May 1, 2017. https://www.nytimes.com/2017/05/01/well/family/for-families-of-teens-at-suicide-risk-13-reasons-triggers-concerns.html.

Scharff, Christina. "Gender and Neoliberalism: Young Women as Ideal Neoliberal Subjects." In *The Handbook of Neoliberalism*, edited by Simon Spring, Kean Birch, and Julie MacLeavy, 217–26. London: Routledge, 2016a.

Scharff, Christina. "The Psychic Life of Neoliberalism: Mapping the Contours of Entrepreneurial Subjectivity." *Theory, Culture & Society* 33, no. 6 (2016b): 107–22. https://doi.org/10.1177/0263276415590164.

Schrodt, Paul. "Lana Del Rey's Feminist Problem." *Slant Magazine*, February 8, 2012. https://www.slantmagazine.com/music/lana-del-reys-feminist-problem/.

Schuster, Sarah. "How Fans Are Showing Demi Lovato She Can Still Be a Role Model After Her Relapse." *The Mighty*, July 27, 2018. https://themighty.com/2018/07/demi-lovato-addiction-overdose-howdemihashelpedme/.

Scott, Katie. "Selena Gomez Reveals Bipolar Disorder Diagnosis." *Globalnews.Ca*, April 6, 2020. https://globalnews.ca/news/6784029/selena-gomez-bipolar/.

Selzer, Jillian. "Celebrities Who Have Talked about Anxiety." *Insider.Com*, September 19, 2018. https://www.insider.com/celebrities-who-talked-about-anxiety-2018-9.

Shugerman, Emily. "Lana Del Rey: Not A Feminist." *Ms. Magazine*, June 12, 2014. http://msmagazine.com/blog/2014/06/12/lana-del-rey-not-a-feminist/.

Singh, Olivia. "28 Celebrities Who Have Opened up about Their Struggles with Mental Illness." *Insider.Com*, May 24, 2019. https://www.insider.com/celebrities-depression-anxiety-mental-health-awareness-2017-11.

Spanos, Brittany. "'Demi Lovato: Dancing With the Devil': Everything We Learned." *Rolling Stone*, April 6, 2021. https://www.rollingstone.com/music/music-news/demi-lovato-dancing-with-the-devil-everything-we-learned-1142242/.

Stables, Paige. "With Rare Beauty, Selena Gomez Has Rewritten the Script for Start-Ups." *Allure*, February 10, 2022. https://www.allure.com/story/selena-gomez-rare-beauty-impact-interview.

Steptoe, Andrew. *Genius and the Mind: Studies of Creativity and Temperament.* Oxford: Oxford University Press, 1998.

Stutz, Colin. "Demi Lovato Releases Bipolar PSA, Announces Mental Health Listening & Engagement Tour." *Billboard.Com*, August 15, 2014. https://www.billboard.com/articles/columns/pop-shop/6221696/demi-lovato-psa-video-mental-health-listening-engagement-tour.

Tannenbaum, Emily. "30 Celebrities Who Have Opened Up About Depression, Anxiety, and Mental Health." *Elle.Com*, May 31, 2017. https://www.elle.com/culture/celebrities/news/g29945/celebrities-depression-anxiety-mental-health/.

Tonic, Gina. "15 Beauty Vloggers Who Are Open About Mental Illness." *Bustle.Com*, October 9, 2016. https://www.bustle.com/articles/188007-15-beauty-vloggers-who-are-open-about-mental-illness.

Truong, Kimberly. "Brittany Snow Spoke 'Too Early' About Mental Health—But She Doesn't Regret It." *InStyle.Com*, October 17, 2019. https://www.instyle.com/celebrity/brittany-snow-almost-family-interview-2019.

Truschel, Jessica. "10 Actors Open Up About Their Battle with Depression." *Psycom.Net*, March 18, 2019. https://www.psycom.net/depression.central.actors.html.

Eijk, Maggy van. "19 Celebrities Who Have Spoken Out About Their Anxiety." *BuzzFeed*, October 15, 2015. https://www.buzzfeed.com/maggyvaneijk/it-aint-about-the-ass-its-about-the-brain.

Vigier, Catherine. "The Meaning of Lana Del Rey: Pop Culture, Post-Feminism and the Choices Facing Young Women Today." *Zeteo: The Journal of Interdisciplinary Writing*, no. Fall (2012): 1–16.

Vivinetto, Gina. "Selena Gomez Reveals Bipolar Disorder Diagnosis: 'It Doesn't Scare Me.'" *Today.Com*, April 4, 2020. https://www.today.com/popculture/selena-gomez-reveals-bipolar-disorder-diagnosis-t177590.

Vogue.com. "Selena Gomez Breaks Her Silence at the AMAs." *Vogue.Com*, November 20, 2016. https://www.vogue.com/article/selena-gomez-american-music-awards-2016-speech.

Vogue.com. "Selena Gomez Gets Real About Anxiety—And How Therapy Changed Everything." *Vogue.Com*, March 16, 2017. https://www.vogue.com/article/selena-gomez-rehab-therapy-mental-health-depression.

Wagner, Bruce. "Billboard Cover: Lana Del Rey on Why Her Pop Stardom 'Could Easily Not Have Happened.'" *Billboard*, October 22, 2015. https://www.billboard.com/articles/news/cover-story/6737539/lana-del-rey-billboard-cover-pop-stardom-relationships-anxiety.

Wallace, Francesca. "A Complete History of Justin Bieber and Selena Gomez's Relationship." *Vogue Australia*, March 9, 2018. https://www.vogue.com.au/celebrity/news/a-complete-history-of-justin-bieber-and-selena-gomezs-relationship/news-story/a1e98bdb9e1192da9cbeda032771ce9e.

Wang, Emily. "Demi Lovato Hospitalized for Apparent Drug Overdose." *Teen Vogue*, July 25, 2018a. https://www.teenvogue.com/story/demi-lovato-hospital-heroin-overdose.

Wang, Emily. "Selena Gomez Is Taking a Social Media Break." *Teen Vogue*, September 24, 2018b. https://www.teenvogue.com/story/selena-gomez-is-taking-a-social-media-break.

Willen, Claudia. "Selena Gomez and Demi Lovato's Friendship Timeline." *Insider. Com*, April 29, 2020. https://www.insider.com/are-selena-gomez-demi-lovato-still-friends-timeline.

Willis, Jackie, and Jennifer Drysdale. "Selena Gomez Hospitalized For Mental Health: A Timeline of Her Struggles." *Entertainment Tonight*, October 11, 2018. https://www.etonline.com/selena-gomez-hospitalized-for-mental-health-a-timeline-of-her-struggles-87220.

Yagoda, Maria. "Gretchen Rossi, Chrissy Teigen & More Stars Who've Opened Up About Their Struggles with Postpartum Depression." *People.Com*, September 26, 2019a. https://people.com/parents/stars-with-postpartum-depression/.

Yagoda, Maria. "'It's Okay Not to Be Strong Sometimes:' 52 Stars Who've Spoken Out About Their Struggles with Mental Health Issues." *People.Com*, October 23, 2019b. https://people.com/health/stars-who-have-mental-illnesses-mental-health-issues/.

Young, Sarah. "Selena Gomez Opens up about Bipolar Diagnosis for First Time during Instagram Live with Miley Cyrus." *Independent.Co.Uk*, April 4, 2020. https://www.independent.co.uk/life-style/selena-gomez-bipolar-mental-health-miley-cyrus-instagram-live-bright-minded-a9447411.html.

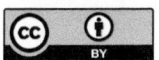

CHAPTER 5

Social Media Sadness: Sad Girl Culture and Radical Ways of Feeling Bad

If you've heard the term "Sad Girl" recently, it's probably in reference to Lana Del Rey, queen of pop melancholy who has inspired a million #PrettyWhenYouCry selfies. It could have been on Tumblr, too, where lately teen angst manifests as dip-dye braids and soft-focus bruises. Actually, when you think about it, Sad Girls are everywhere—in the musings of Twitter personality @SoSadToday, the selfies of artist Audrey Wollen, creator of "Sad Girl Theory," and on Etsy, where you can buy Sad Girl necklaces, pins, vests, and tote bags, typically in pastel.[1]

The above quote is from a 2015 article titled "A taxonomy of the sad girl" in the fashion and style magazine *i-D*, and I include it here because it captures the multifaceted presence of the sad girl online at the time (this magazine also declared 2015 the year of the sad girl).[2] Like other internet phenomena, the sad girl has taken many different forms and cannot be easily pinpointed or narrowed down into one specific thing. This chapter turns to the worlds of social media platforms to understand how mental illness was spoken about in gendered ways online during the 2010s through this figure of the "sad girl," one most broadly defined as "a young woman who is unashamed of her emotional life and who fearlessly acts out her pain for others to see."[3]

Several writers in the smaller popular press (fashion/style magazines that cover internet culture) have written about how she appears on different platforms, describing the kind of posts shared and favored by the sad girls on Tumblr and Instagram[4] as well as covered specific prolific sad girls like artist Audrey Wollen,[5] writer Melissa Broder (@sosadtoday on Twitter)[6]

© The Author(s) 2023
F. Thelandersson, *21st Century Media and Female Mental Health*,
https://doi.org/10.1007/978-3-031-16756-0_5

and the collective Sad Girls Club.[7] Attention has also been given to the fashion trends of wearing your mental distress on your sleeve, so to speak, with hats declaring "being sad is ok," sweatshirts reading "emotional tendencies," and a brand called "Cry Baby" which has the tagline "i made this brand to show you that it's okay to cry."[8]

So far the scholarly study of the sad girl has been limited. Several journal articles have been written about the presence of content depicting non-suicidal self-injury (NSSI) in online contexts, primarily from a health care perspective that looks at how Internet spaces encourage or discourage self-injury.[9] There have also been a few studies from a media studies perspective about specific online forums for mental health support like Ian Tucker and Lewis Goodings' examination of the UK based site *Elefriends* or Anthony McCosker's analysis of the Australian mental health organization *beyondblue*, both of which point to the importance of social media and peer influencers in the treatment and recovery from mental illness.[10] Among those who have focused specifically on the sad girl are Eileen Mary Holowka, who has written about the way the sad girls of Instagram function as a community and a counter public, and Heather Mooney who has examined the racial aspects of the sad girl in comparison to another affective figure circulating online, the Carefree Black Girl.[11]

It is important to note in the discussion of sad girls that even if this figure was at its most visible online during 2014-2015, that iteration of the figure could be said to have originated in the Chicana/Latina culture of 1990s Los Angeles. One of the groups I look at in this chapter, Mexico-based Sad Girls Y Qué, explicitly traces the use of the term to this context and calls out other sad girls for ignoring these roots. I do not, however, see this as a simple case of cultural appropriation, following an understanding of the term as one involving cultural exploitation and disrespect.[12] It is rather a case of a range of sources influencing a particular cultural expression, and the multiple inspirations behind the figure of the sad girl show the fluidity of cultural sharing and creativity in a digital world. I discuss the specific aspects of this later in the chapter.

Zoe Alderton, from whom I borrow the broad definition of the sad girl mentioned above, has done a meticulous job of studying the visual rhetoric of online self-harm communities and dedicates an entire chapter of her book *The Aesthetics of Self-Harm* to sad girls and "the internet and the performance of mood."[13] Alderton notes that the #sadgirl tag on Tumblr contains images of self-harm and suicidal ideation but also involves "a high degree of self-awareness," noting that "while the sadness is genuine, performances are often overblown or ironic."[14] This distance and irony are key to understanding the sad girl phenomenon, and by taking these aspects into account one can move away from a simple "good" or "bad" value judgment about young people's practice of sharing dark feelings online, which is often the case in the scholarly pieces from researchers with roots in medical fields. Alderton's approach is more nuanced as she notes that:

> The Sad Girl is core to a new brand of feminism and philosophy that defines the performance of mood online, revealing both *why* young women are so sad and *how* sadness can actually be a way of releasing negative affect and protesting wrongdoing rather than wallowing in non-action.[15]

I follow this approach in my examination of the sad girl phenomenon as I hope to be able to open up discussion toward questions about whether or not the sad girls are sharing a new kind of sadness, and if so, in what ways this might challenge traditional conceptions of sadness and mental illness. While the previous two chapters dealt with more conventional types of media and popular culture, this chapter turns to the world of Internet peer-to-peer networks and smaller micro-celebrities to examine how mental health was talked about there.

This chapter also further opens up the connections between mental illness and sadness. In the previous chapter I traced the links between Selena Gomez's mental health advocacy, her use of sad aesthetics in her work, and Lana del Rey's embracement of a sad persona. In the analysis of sad girls on social media, the connection between sadness and mental health continues as I consider not only mentions of specific diagnoses but also general sad feelings like isolation, despair, abandonment issues, and general disaffectedness.

In what follows I discuss how the sad girl appeared on the social media platforms Tumblr and Instagram, and the specific cases of Audrey Wollen, Sad Girls Y Qué, Sad Girls Club, and My Therapist Says. These cases are all examples of various ways of sharing one's disaffected/negative feelings online, some explicitly adopting the label sad girl and others only writing about feeling bad. There is a spectrum of peer vs. hierarchical groups here, where some figurations see most users more or less equal to each other in terms of follower counts and others take the form of a few micro-celebrities posting to a large number of followers. This spectrum can be identified by platform. On Tumblr, users were fairly equalized due to the distributed forms of posting and reblogging (more on that below), whereas on

Instagram the networks were structured more around a few influential users with large followings who obtain micro-celebrity status. Additionally, there were differences between the various micro-celebrities, where someone like Audrey Wollen inhabits an activist and art-oriented position compared to the more business-oriented profile of the account My Therapist Says. I discuss these differences and the critical and acritical tendencies in the sad girl figure, as well as the themes of relatability, impasse, dynamics of coping, suffering, and normalization's ambivalence. I explore how the Tumblr sad girls can be read as playing with the potential of impasse and resting in sadness by refusing to work immediately toward a cure, whereas their counterparts on Instagram are often explicitly political. I also consider the various levels of support found among the different versions of sad girls and how they navigate the display yet disavowal of injuries. Humor is a recurring aspect of the social media accounts I discuss here, both as a form of coping and a way to create community through "shared literacies."[16] This chapter also argues that some of the sad girls are examples of the kind of "precarity-focused consciousness raising" proposed by the *Institute for Precarious Consciousness.*

The "feeling rules" of neoliberalism and the notion of relatability are common threads in this chapter. Gill and Kanai point to the social "feeling rules" (after Hochschild) of neoliberalism, of which the "confidence cult" and the relatable self are two integral parts of how women especially are urged to express their feelings.[17] They argue that this joint imperative to confidence and relatability put women in a "double bind" in which they have to be "'relatable' but 'confident' in the appropriate proportions."[18] Throughout this chapter I look at how various manifestations of sad girls and other discussions of depression, anxiety, and "feeling bad" are expressed in relatable and not-so-relatable ways.

And again, these sad girls exist within the confidence culture outlined by Orgad and Gill, where the tendency by female subjects to share vulnerable moments largely is a move to appear authentic and relatable.[19] Even though this is the larger media culture in which the figure of the sad girl emerged, and some of the figure's iterations are of the lightheartedly relatable kind, I argue that something else is happening in the expression of the negative here. Whereas the vulnerability expressed in the confidence culture is one that has already been overcome,[20] the feelings of despair and anxiety expressed by sad girls are often shared as they happen. The expressions of mental illness and sadness discussed in the previous chapters are largely examples of a profitable vulnerability while the sad girl culture explored here opens up more spacious ways of feeling bad.

Affective Resonance

Anna Gibbs uses the term "affective resonance" to designate how affects are spread and taken up among different individuals. She defines this as "the positive feedback loops created by affect, and in particular to the tendency of someone witnessing the display of affect in another person to resonate with and experience the same affect in response."[21] In other words, when seeing someone else express a particular affect the chances are high that you will also adopt that affect. Among "sad girls" on the social media platforms I discuss in this chapter, the sharing of affective content by individual users resonates with other users and together form a mutual "sad girl affect," specific to each platform and sub-group of users. Gibbs writes that "repeated experiences of affective resonance (whether 'firsthand' or 'mediated') produce a concatenation in which affect resonates with like affect, so as to link otherwise unrelated scenes without producing articulable meaning."[22] The repetition of the sad girl affect in a recurring affective resonance creates a shared "sad girl aesthetic" whose meaning cannot be directly explained, but makes sense to the sad girls who participate in its creation and maintenance.

Taking it one step further, it can also be suggested that it is not just an affect and aesthetic that is being disseminated, but also a subjective figure of the sad girl. Jack Bratich has studied the memes generated around and out of the Occupy Wall Street (OWS) movement to gain "insight into its mediated subjective processes." He explains that "OWS started as a meme by meme specialists and then mutated into a meme-generator, flashmob, and platform."[23] Bratich defines OWS as a potential aggregator of subjectivities, arguing that the movement "could be a name for an aggregate of operations, even an emergent subjective figure."[24] I think it can be helpful to think of the figure of the sad girl as constituting a similar "mediated subjective process." Through the sharing and reblogging of affective images, the subject position of the sad girl emerges and becomes available for users to inhabit. Via meme-tic sharing of content, a shared experience of sadness is formed within the online communities of sad girls.

Tumblr Sad Girls

Tumblr started in 2007 as a microblogging and social networking site.[25] The site established a reputation among the major social media sites as "a comfortable place to be honest, weird, and maybe even depressed"[26] and scholars have identified it as particularly conducive for LGBTQIA+ communities and niche fandoms.[27] It differs from other social media platforms in a few significant ways: it functions more like a blog than other social media sites, the content posted is published to each user's own Tumblr page which is visible also to nonusers (the design of this page can be endlessly modified, something I elaborate on below). The social aspects of Tumblr resemble other platforms in a few ways: users follow each other via linear news feeds like that on Facebook, Instagram, or Twitter; one can post original content in the form of text, image, quote, link, chat, audio, and video; and one can reblog or like someone else's posts. Much of the content that circulates among the sad girls has been reblogged thousands of times. This number is trackable in a "notes"-section found at the bottom of each post, each note representing one reblog or like. Study of the phenomenon of the sad girl on Tumblr cannot include only an examination of a few users' original content, but needs to follow the content that is being spread in a meme-like fashion on the site.

Something to note in relation to all of the iterations of sad girls discussed in this chapter is the role of platform politics and technological affordances. Bryce Renninger points out in his study of counter publics on Tumblr that "with changes in platforms and networks of users, media ideologies shift."[28] Such shifts contribute to the move of users from one platform to another, or the "spreading out" of activity across multiple platforms. The popularity of Tumblr has shifted since the beginning of the time period that I am examining.[29] At the time of writing Tumblr is still up and running, but many of the sad girl accounts that I follow are no longer active on the platform. Nevertheless, the Tumblr sad girl activity that I discuss here was a big part of the site during the time period of 2013–2017.

On Tumblr, some typical examples of content circulated by sad girls are pictures of pills in bright pink colors; animated texts that read things like "having a threesome with anxiety and depression"; glittering words that spell out "100% Sad" (see Fig. 5.1); and cartoon character Lisa Simpson lying face down on her bed with the word sad girl spelled out in the front and center of the image.[30]

Posts like these position sadness and depression as a shared and common experience. Statements like "having a threesome with anxiety and depression" do not portray anxiety and depression as by default negative ailments to be cured; neither does it position them as something to be ashamed of. Instead it states loud and clear that the person posting it is

Fig. 5.1 100% Sad, Tumblr post by Less-love-more-alcohol, source: Thelandersson, "Social Media Sad Girls and the Normalization of Sad States of Being"

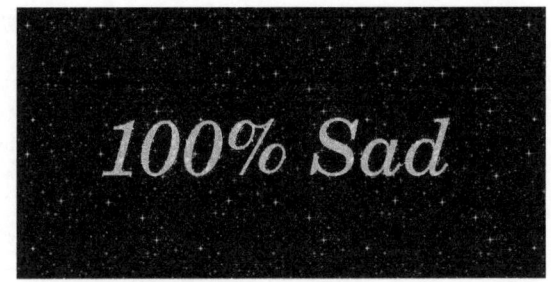

living with anxiety and depression, and has come to terms with it enough to formulate the suffering in a distanced way. One post about psychotropic drugs depicts pink pills in a polaroid-like frame with the word "Medicated" written at the bottom (see Fig. 5.2). Another is just a picture of a pile of turquoise pills with the imprint "S 90 3."[31] A simple google search for this code reveals that the drug portrayed is the benzodiazepine Xanax. Posts like these both normalize and glorify psychopharmacology. There are also those that communicate the commonness of therapy, like a photograph of a framed poster that spells out "I told my therapist about you."[32]

The archive I draw on here is not a fixed or limited set of Tumblr accounts, but rather content I have seen circulated multiple times among the sad girls I follow on the site. I have been an observer of Tumblr since early 2010 and have tracked the emerging sad girl content on the site, which led me to follow the accounts that were most active in posting about these kinds of topics.

I have paid particular attention to the posts with a high number of notes, or reblogs. Due to its technological affordances like pseudonyms and modifiable HTML, Tumblr lends itself to a sad girl aesthetic.[33] The majority of these users do not use their real names, as is common practice on many other social media sites. This allows for a more open sharing of personal experiences and feelings that people in their everyday lives might find alarming, "abnormal," or shameful. Several of the sad girls have also taken full advantage of the modifiable HTML, creating elaborately designed banners, including moving glitter backgrounds and gifs that reveal more information as you scroll over them.[34] For example, user Grvnge-nicotine has a header that shows a picture of Uma Thurman in Pulp Fiction smoking a cigarette, displayed on a background of crystals and pink pills. Surrounding, and on top of, this image are phrases like "I hate everything," "anti-you," and "you little shit" in various figurations

Fig. 5.2 "Medicated," Tumblr post by Grvnge-nicotine, source: Thelandersson, "Social Media Sad Girls and the Normalization of Sad States of Being"

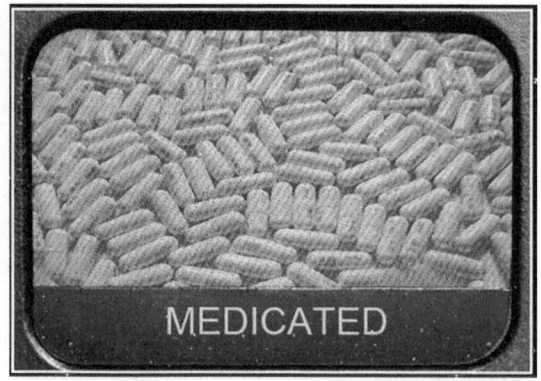

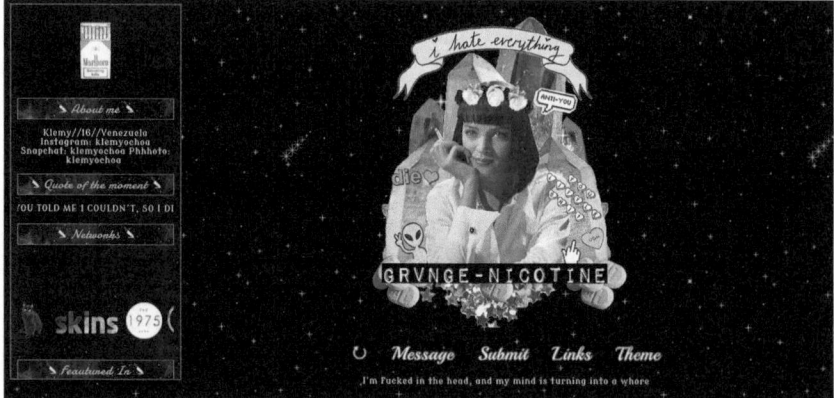

Fig. 5.3 Banner of Tumblr user Grvnge-nicotine, source: Thelandersson, "Social Media Sad Girls and the Normalization of Sad States of Being"

and colors. In the top left corner of her site is a spinning pack of Marlboro cigarettes, which, if you hover over it, reveals informational blurbs under the headings "About me," "Quote of the moment," "Networks," and "Featured in" (see Fig. 5.3).

When one scrolls down the page, the posts made by Grvnge-nicotine are seen in chronological order, with the newest on top. This is the way most sad girls design their Tumblr blogs, and it shows their posts lined up together in about five columns, creating a larger compositional image that conveys a shared sad girl aesthetic by displaying several of their posts together at the same time (see Fig. 5.4).

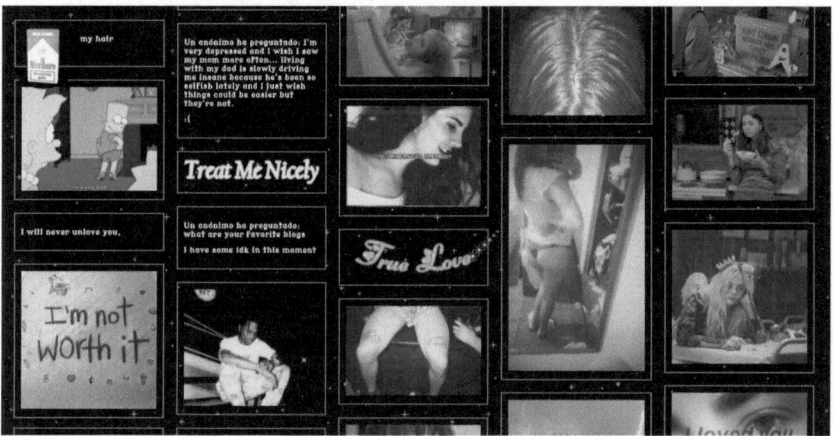

Fig. 5.4 Compilation of posts on the Tumblr account of user Grvnge-nicotine, source: Thelandersson, "Social Media Sad Girls and the Normalization of Sad States of Being"

Suffering as Ordinary

Lisa Blackman's notion of "reframing suffering as 'ordinary'" becomes relevant here.[35] She explains that conceiving "suffering as 'ordinary'" reframes it as "not an exceptional phenomenon, but rather part and parcel of the costs of neo-liberalism(s)."[36] By conceptualizing suffering as ordinary, one can acknowledge the "difficulties of living normalised fictions and fantasies of femininity that [are] produced within [neoliberalism(s)] ... as signs of personal failure, inadequacy and the associated economies of pain, fear, anxiety and distress that keep these apparatuses alive and in place."[37] Seeing suffering as ordinary, and not something that can immediately be cured or done away with, makes it possible to connect suffering with the neoliberal power structures that control our wellbeing while telling us that we have endless possibilities to maximize our mental and physical health. The sad girls on Tumblr do seem to see suffering as ordinary, as they rest in it as a part of everyday life that they cannot get away from. For example, a post by user straightboyfriend that has been reblogged and liked 42,304 times reads "its summer vacation you know what that means! Isolation & severe depression."[38] Another post, by user gothicprep, which has been reblogged and liked 58,058 times, reads "how do i contour my abandonment issues?"[39] Both posts imply a base level of constant sadness, and the ironic tone serves to establish shared connections with other users who have had similar experiences. The connection of sad feelings (isolation, severe depression, and abandonment issues) with usually joyful and "normal" things (summer vacation and makeup) turns the negative feelings into a shared comedic discourse.

Coping Through Humor

Within psychology, humor has long been acknowledged as a coping mechanism that can ease an individual's experiences of stressful events. Freud regarded it to be the highest form of defense mechanism, arguing that "the essence of humor is that one spares oneself the affects to which the situation would naturally give rise and overrides with a jest the possibility of such an emotional display."[40] Later theorists have praised the humorist's ability for "rapid perceptual-cognitive switches in frames of reference,"[41] which creates a distance that removes the individual "from the immediate threat, of a problem situation, to view it from a different perspective, and, therefore, to reduce the often paralyzing feelings of anxiety and helplessness."[42] Within this reasoning around humor, the jokes shared by the Tumblr sad girls can be interpreted as signs that this online discourse gives the individual users participating in it a relief from their immediate problems and difficult feelings. Studies about how humor is being implemented by various individuals have, however, somewhat complicated this notion of humor as a coping mechanism. Rod A. Martin and Herbert M. Lefcourt, for example, found that humor does reduce the impact of stress, but for it to do so, "the individual must also place a high value on humor and, more importantly, produce humor, particularly in the stressful situations that he or she encounters in daily life."[43] Later, Martin and his students developed the Humor Styles Questionnaire to assess how individuals use humor in their daily lives,[44] which has been used in hundreds of studies within the field of psychology since.[45] The questionnaire gives individuals scores on four different styles of humor: affiliative (use of humor to "enhance one's relationships with others"), self-enhancing ("relatively benign uses of humor to enhance the self"), aggressive ("use of humor to enhance the self at the expense of others"), and self-defeating ("use of humor to enhance relationships at the expense of self").[46] Scoring high on the first two (positive) humor styles has been linked to positive health outcomes, such as "being happier and having healthier relationships," whereas having high scores on the last two (negative) styles have been linked to negative effects on health.[47] A 2019 study using the questionnaire found that people diagnosed with depression used self-defeating humor more than nondepressed people, and that depressive individuals used the two positive humor styles (affiliative and self-enhancing) less than non-depressive individuals.[48] The relation between humor and wellbeing, then, is more nuanced than simply "humor eases suffering and stress," and self-defeating humor can in some cases be signs of worsening (or unchanged) mental illness issues. But the examples from the Tumblr sad girls mentioned above can also be read as examples of affiliative humor that enhances the relationships among the peers participating in the discussion, by joking about the conditions of living with depression and anxiety that they all share.

The use of humor in online contexts has been analyzed by feminist media studies scholars as a means of creating "shared literacies"[49] in digital spaces, with feminist memes in particular being marked as tools to create "online spaces of consciousness raising and community building."[50] I will discuss the politically inflected community building aspects of feminist humor in online spaces more below, in relation to the sad girls on Instagram, for whom comedy and memes are a more central aspect of their online activities.

Impasse: Acedia and Melancholia

Blackman and Ann Cvetkovich have written about the "productive possibilities of negative states of being," which seek to "to de-pathologise shame, melancholy, failure, depression, anxieties and other forms of 'feeling bad,' to open up new ways of thinking about agency, change and transformation."[51] Cvetkovich describes how the Public Feelings project uses the term impasse to refer to "a state of both stuckness and potential."[52] She explains that the notion of impasse maintains "a hopefulness about the possibility that slowing down or not moving forward might not be a sign of failure and might instead be worth exploring."[53] Impasse could be one kind of productive possibility, allowing sufferers to rest in "bad" feelings without having to immediately work to get rid of them. Similar to Blackman's notion of suffering as ordinary,[54] the concept of impasse allows us to think about and process the power structures that inevitably affect the possibilities of succeeding at a healthy life. Among the sad girls on Tumblr, there is usually not an overt political engagement that directly connects suffering to structures of power. But the mere act of resting in sadness, as they do, might function as an impasse, where the refusal to move forward becomes a protest of the neoliberal demands of becoming a laboring and "happy" subject. Examples of this kind of resting in sadness include a glittering GIF that spells out "Self-destructive and unproductive," a picture of a white t-shirt with the text "I've Been Crying All Day" accompanied by a red rose, and a fake resume that includes items like "Battled Depression 2000-2013."[55] Posts like these present a kind of opposite to the neoliberal feminism that urges women to "lean in" to competitive work environments, and can instead be read as encouraging the reader to "lean in" to nonaction, self-destructiveness, and sadness.

Two terms that can describe the kind of resting in sadness performed by the sad girls on Tumblr are acedia and melancholia. Acedia, first mentioned in early Christian writings on monastic life, refers to spiritual crisis, inertia, carelessness, and intense feelings of disgust and disdain.[56] The term has generally been considered too religious to be used in understanding contemporary depression. But Cvetkovich argues that "acedia helps place the medical model of depression within the longer history of notions of not only health but embodiment of what it means to be human."[57] Thinking of depression as an "embodiment of what it means to be human" implies a rejection of a medical model that sees depression as something exceptional to be immediately cured away, and instead assigns it a central place in the experience of life itself. The tendency to conceive of depression as abnormal indirectly marks "feeling good" as the "normal" mood for which one should always aim.

Adopting a model of acedia that places depression as central to what it means to be human, allows a move away from seeing it as exceptional. Instead, it can be viewed as something that offers an opportunity to pause and break from the requirement to constantly be a profit-making subject, and provide a chance to process the emotional impacts of life under neoliberalism. In their refusal to heal, the sad girls can perhaps be an example of conceptualizing sadness as acedia.

Besides accepting sadness as ordinary, the sad girls on Tumblr can also be read as displaying an idealization of sadness. This could be described by the concept of melancholia, which has also been used as an alternative to contemporary medical models. Cvetkovich explains that melancholia allows for "a return to a time when sadness could be viewed in other ways, including as a normative part of cultural experience, and even, most notably in the case of Renaissance and Romantic understandings that have had a persistent influence, as a creative force."[58] It is something that touches more upon sadness in general, a sadness that is creative and inspiring, rather than the debilitating "stuck-ness" associated with depression.

There is also an element of pleasure in melancholia. Freudian psychoanalysis defines the melancholic as "one who incorporates a lost object of desire into her ego, so that she never fully experiences the loss, since the loved one, even in absence, becomes merged with the self."[59] The lost love becomes integral to the make-up of the subject, to her entire self-image, and the incorporation of the loss takes the form of masochistic pleasure in love relationships. The pleasurable and creative aspect of melancholia differs significantly from the spiritual crisis and inertia of acedia. I think one can hold on to both concepts as ways of thinking through depression and sadness.

In relation to the sad girls on Tumblr, melancholia can capture the pleasure they derive in glorifying sadness, and acedia the inertia that co-exists with this romanticizing. Melancholia might be said to glorify feeling bad because of its promise to produce great art; it is the driving force of the archetypical tortured genius. In this way, the sad girls seem to partially adhere to a melancholic stance. There is a dedication to artists and celebrities that fulfill this role of tortured and misunderstood genius. Lana del Rey is the most frequently occurring figure in this context. The sad girls on Tumblr adopt her affect by posting and reblogging images of her, sometimes with lyrics from her songs written on them. She even has a song entitled "Sad Girl" that contains the lyrics "I'm a sad girl, I'm a bad girl, I'm a bad girl." Another popular del Rey lyric that is repeatedly reblogged is "you like your girls insane," from the song "Born to Die," shared as text atop a photograph of the singer.[60] del Rey and the persona she inhabits (see discussion in the previous chapter) lends herself perfectly to the Tumblr sad girl aesthetic, shown by the frequency with which images of her and her songs are reblogged and spread among these Tumblr users.

Idealizations of real-life persons who inhabit the position of (female) misinterpreted and tortured genius are also common. The trainwreck celebrities discussed in Chap. 4 appear here as revered figures. Courtney Love, Amy Winehouse, Sky Ferreira, and celebrities who have had public breakdowns, like Britney Spears, Lindsey Lohan, and Amanda Bynes seem to reinforce a melancholic notion of sadness as romantic, mystical, and inspirational.[61] Acedia and melancholia are ways of conceptualizing sadness beyond the pro- or anti- medical model offered by psychiatry. I believe these concepts can explain the activity of the sad girls by providing ways of thinking about the simultaneous resting in, and normalizing of, sadness and the glorification of feeling bad.

A Supportive Community?

It is in the collective notions of sadness that develop among the sad girls on Tumblr, that the alternative conceptualizations of sadness move from theoretical to actual. By sharing their own views of sadness on this platform, it becomes possible for Tumblr sad girls to explore their feelings together, and potentially provide support for one another by validating each other's experiences. The glorification of sadness found among the sad girls here sometimes borders on the encouragement of self-destructive behavior. But, paradoxically, the fact that these experiences are shared within the virtual space intervenes in the glorified isolation and presents the possibility of a supportive collective. On Tumblr, in the middle of del Rey quotes and pictures of pills, more "positive" posts are found. For example, a gif of moving text that reads "sext: I want to be good for your mental health."[62] "Sext" refers to the communication of sexual acts via text message, or, the text version of phone sex. "Sext:" followed by various sentences is a meme that juxtaposes the sexual connotations of "sexting" with nonsexual phrases for comedic effect. Saying "I want to be good for your mental health" in this context communicates a tender longing for emotional support and stability. This speaks to the complexities and nuances of the normalizing discourse happening here. On the one hand, there is a risk of glorifying/getting stuck, but in the very act of sharing one learns that one is not alone and a kind of community is created.

AUDREY WOLLEN: SAD GIRL THEORY

One of the most highly publicized sad girls was the artist Audrey Wollen, who in 2014 gained widespread attention and media coverage with her "Sad Girl Theory." Wollen's artistic practice took place largely on Instagram, where she would post images of herself looking sad, often with smudged makeup in the middle of crying and tagging it #sadgirl.[63] There was also a series of photos recreating famous classical paintings but with details from modern girlhood, like a recreation of Diego Velázquez's 1651 painting *The Rokeby Venus*. In the original painting, Venus lies naked on a bed, with her back to the viewer and looking at a reflection of herself in a mirror being held up by a kneeling cherub. In Wollen's version, the artist herself lies in the same position as Venus, naked and with her back turned to the viewer, staring at a laptop computer perched on a small table.[64] Wollen also posted multiple photos of herself posing in doctor's offices, undressed in examination rooms where she went to get treatment for her chronic illness.[65] For Wollen this was not merely an expression of her own feelings and experiences, but a political act on a larger scale. She describes the theory behind it as follows:

> Sad Girl Theory is the proposal that the sadness of girls should be witnessed and re-historicized as an act of resistance, of political protest. Basically, girls being sad has been categorized as this act of passivity, and therefore, discounted from the history of activism. I'm trying to open up the idea that protest doesn't have to be external to the body; it doesn't have to be a huge march in the streets, noise, violence, or rupture. There's a long history of girls who have used their own anguish, their own suffering, as tools for resistance and political agency. Girls' sadness isn't quiet, weak, shameful, or dumb: It is active, autonomous, and articulate. It's a way of fighting back.[66]

In this way Wollen directly politicized the sad girl and put her expression of suffering onto a larger scale. In interviews Wollen expressed discomfort with "the hyper-positive demands of contemporary feminism" that is fixated on self-love, approval, and "making it cool and fun to be a girl."[67] The problem with this, for Wollen, is that "it isn't really cool and fun to be a girl. It is an experience of brutal alienation and constant fear of violence."[68] Here Wollen indirectly marks out the "feeling rules" of the contemporary moment for women and girls that Gill and Kanai write about in relation to neoliberalism and postfeminism, and of which the "confidence cult" is an integral part.[69]

Wollen's work was widely covered in smaller popular press outlets and art magazines like *Dazed Digital*, *NYLON*, *i-D*, and *Artillery* magazine, and from 2014 to early 2016 it seemed like she was everywhere on this part of the Internet.[70] In the art magazine *Artillery*, Emily Wells pointed specifically to Wollen's claim of sadness as "an inherent threat to the status quo of oppression" which Wells saw Wollen doing by "challenging the hyper-positive, self-love-or-nothing feminism that permeates the Internet, and alienates feminists who are unable to subscribe to it."[71] This commentary on Wollen's work might betray why she received so much attention, that is, because at the time, the feminism most visible in popular culture was one of empowerment and strength, and the notion that feminism could embrace a language of weakness seemed truly radical.

In interviews Wollen also mentioned singer Lana del Rey as an example of a sad girl (alongside historical figures like the writer Virginia Woolf and the saint St Catherine of Siena) and praised her performative displays of sadness.[72] And as discussed in the introduction and in the celebrity chapter, del Rey can also be read as a response to an overtly positive feminism that does not leave any room for suffering. Alderton sees in del Rey someone who not only "represents narratives of female weakness, sadness, and failure" but also "speaks to a generation who feel cut out of their forebears' market economy."[73] For Alderton, Wollen and del Rey are on the same continuum of sad girls that display sadness and weakness that represents women on a larger scale. I agree with this argument and the notion that the popularity of both del Rey and Wollen speaks to the frustrations of women at the time. These frustrations were first expressed among del Rey's fans and in the subcultural public online spaces that Wollen inhabited, and later appeared also in a broader popular culture as seen by the increase in celebrity confessions and the turn to sadness in pop music, culminating in the rise of Billie Eilish in 2019 (as discussed in Chap. 4).

Wollen received largely positive media coverage and gained a following of 25,000 on Instagram, which made her into a kind of micro-celebrity. But her role as an artist and feminist activist put her in a different position than the micro-celebrities usually associated with this platform, which tend to be "conventionally good-looking or people who display status symbols like luxury goods, due to the app's focus on visuals."[74] Wollen fits more into the category of subcultural or niche micro-celebrity, who have large amounts of followers but remain unknown to the larger public and are largely ignored by mainstream media.[75]

In early 2016 Wollen posted an image of her iPhone next to a white lily, the phone screen displaying a sad-looking selfie of the artist herself. In a lengthy caption she announced that she had decided to take a hiatus from social media, explaining that she had become "increasingly unsettled and at times deeply hurt by the climate of online feminism" and her position within it.[76] She expressed discomfort specifically in relation to her political intentions and the ways they had been misconstrued on the platform:

> … i worry my ideas are eclipsed by my identity as an "instagram girl" and i watch as ppl whose work i really respect write me off and ppl whose work i don't respect cite me as inspiration. "sad girl theory" is often understood at its most reductive, instead of as a proposal to open up more spacious discussions abt what activism could look like. my internet presence has been the best and worst thing in my life, and i owe it so much (so many friends! so much knowledge! so much solidarity and hope!!!) and i also find myself afraid of it, afraid of fucking up, afraid of being misunderstood, afraid of trusting ppl…[77]

Wollen's doubts and her reasons for leaving Instagram speak to the problems of cultivating activism on corporate platforms that value interaction in the form of likes and comments, which often reduces nuanced messages to bite-sized and easily digestible content. Wollen did not delete her account, however; instead it lay dormant up until February 2019, when she removed most of her old posts (including the ones about Sad Girl Theory) and tentatively started posting again.[78] This speaks to the impermanence of social media platforms and how fickle internet phenomena can be. What remains available of Wollen's work is the writing about it by journalists and writers in other outlets.

Wollen's changed relationship with Instagram also speaks to the role of technological affordances of the social media platform being used. When I was trying to find out what had happened to Wollen and her work I found an article in *VICE*, titled "Remembering Instagram Before the Influencers" published in July 2019. In it the writer mentions Wollen alongside other young artists who were popular on Instagram in the mid-2010s but who now have different relationships with the platform. One of them says about the early days of Instagram (which launched in 2010) that it "wasn't so censored ... it felt more DIY and achievable. It wasn't so algorithm-heavy. I felt like it was more efficient. Whereas now, it feels like you have to invest money and do sponsored posts."[79] This refers partly to the change in the platform's algorithm, which went from showing users a chronological news feed of posts to one ordered by Instagram's secret mechanisms that privilege ads and sponsored posts. This is a reminder that users of corporate platforms like Tumblr and Instagram are always at the mercy of the corporate owners for whom profit-making is the ultimate incentive. Changes to the platform affordances such as the algorithm of the news feed that determines how many of your followers will actually see your posts can affect both individual users' engagement and larger trends in who uses what platforms.

Sad Girls Y Qué: The (Presumed) Whiteness of the Sad Girl

Sad Girls Y Qué was another group that emerged online in 2014. Based out of Tijuana, Mexico, they described themselves as a "glittery, girl power gang" that used Internet art "to retaliate against the culture of machismo prevalent in Mexico and the world at large while reappropriating a girly 'feminine' aesthetic." Run by five Chicana-identified women, the group mainly used a "Tumblr-style Facebook page" to curate images of "alternative icons like Selena [Quintanilla Pérez], animated characters like Sailor Moon, and sex-positive imagery" as well as post "heartbreak poems and notes on depression and solitude."[80,81]

For Sad Girls Y Qué the figure of the sad girl comes from the Chola culture represented in the 1993 film *Mi Vida Loca*, which takes place in Los Angeles (at the time Latinx-dominated) neighborhood Echo Park. In this context the sad girl comes from LA tattoo art where she is seen as "a gangster chick with tears running down her face." Importantly "this image of a crying woman is not a weak victim. She's tough and conveys a more complex range of femininity."[82] An early definition of the sad girl on the site Urban Dictionary, which crowdsources definitions of emerging vernacular, confirms this origin of the figure: "A nickname that is Chicana/Latina in origin, Sad Girl usually refers to a tough girl who has suffered extreme hardships."[83]

In an interview with *VICE* magazine Anna Bon, one of the members, defines the sad girl as "any girl who is fed up with society's standards and patriarchy" but specifies that the figure comes from Chicana culture. Bon's definition of the sad girl here is different than the broader one laid out by Alderton, which I cite at the beginning of this chapter. This exemplifies the differences within the figure and the fluidity of the concept, showing how the same term may mean different things to different groups. For Bon and Sad Girls Y Qué, ignoring the Latinx origins of the sad girl amounts to a whitewashing of the concept. In the interview with *VICE* Bon indirectly calls out Wollen (who went to California Institute of the Arts, or CalArts, at the time), saying "There's this group of artists in LA who call themselves 'sad girls' and they're all white girls from CalArts. It's cool that the sad girl term is a trend and a thing, but the appropriation of it is annoying and offensive."[84] This speaks not only to Wollen and her sad girl theory, but also to the stereotypical sad girl as someone who has relied primarily on "white bodies as a way of presenting depressive themes and exploring girlhood."[85] In her analysis of sad girls and the figure of the Black Carefree Girl, Mooney notes that the sad girl sometimes uses aesthetics from Latina/x culture in ways that constitute cultural appropriation. She points to Lana del Rey's 2013 video Tropico, a short film in which the singer wears clothes reminiscent of the Virgin Mary and works as a stripper in Los Angeles as an example.[86] Mooney notes that del Rey is repeatedly shown "inhaling the smoke exhaled by her Latina/x consort …

[she] 'breathes in' racialized space and embodied 'authenticity,' animating her position as a 'real' Sad Girl. The narrative and surroundings are presented as objects, consumable by Del Rey and her viewers."[87]

For Mooney the sad girl manages to resist the "affective hegemony of white girlhood" by showing the "failure of normative empowerment models" and the "problems with can-do girlhood."[88] But the resistance expressed here will always be limited by the fact that the sad girl is "a product of cultural appropriation and neoliberalism, and the affective legacies of whiteness contour her emergence."[89] It is important to note these differences and tensions in the sad girl before too easily embracing her as a subversive alternative to an upbeat popular feminism, as in Wollen's rendering of sadness as protest. Mooney's positioning of the sad girl in relation to can-do girlhood is instructive when thinking about the racialized aspects of the figure. Even if the can-do girl is not exclusively white, whiteness is an important aspect of can-do girlhood, and white images of sad girlhood risk positioning only white girls as able to resist the demands of can-do-ness. Mooney's critique here also suggests that the release that can be found in fully giving in to sadness/adopting a sad girl position/identity, as Wollen's sad girl theory proposes, is mostly available to white women and girls, as they are the ones that the empowerment discourse of can-do-ness and popular feminism is aimed at. I believe one way of doing these tensions justice, is to ask who gets to inhabit the position of unashamedly displaying their sadness online. As I briefly discussed in the previous chapter, the celebrities who have been the most vocal and visible about their mental illnesses are white or white-passing, indicating the limitations of that position. Among the sad girls on Tumblr, when images of bodies appear they tend to be white and thin, suggesting that inhabiting positions of acedia and melancholia are mostly available to white girls and women. The work of the Sad Girls Club on Instagram, which I will discuss further below, directly addresses this issue by focusing specifically on women of color suffering from mental illness.

INSTAGRAM SAD GIRLS

Wollen was not the last sad girl on Instagram, however, and from 2016 and onward, a group of users on the platform gained large followings through posting about their mental distress in humorous ways. The design and affordances of Instagram are more static than Tumblr, with all users of the platform having a fixed profile that always displays the number of followers that a particular user has. This makes the activity on the site more centralized than on Tumblr, with a few users emerging as the most influential in terms of how many followers they display on their profile and how many likes their individual posts get.[90]

Studying the sad girls of Instagram thus becomes a look at the most popular accounts and the kind of content they share, in contrast to the sad girls of Tumblr among which posts are shared and spread multiple times in larger numbers. Although Instagram users do repost each other at times, this practice is not at all as widespread as the reblogging on Tumblr, where content is spread faster than on Instagram.

Among the sad girls on Instagram, the most popular accounts were generally focused on making fun of mental distress through memes and other comedic portrayals. Astrology, leftist politics, and the disappointment of heterosexual men were also popular topics.[91] The users who gained the most followers obtained a sort of micro-celebrity status, but as discussed above in relation to Wollen, the content for which they are known puts them more in the position of subcultural or niche micro-celebrity compared to the conventionally good-looking and luxury-focused micro-celebrities usually associated with Instagram.[92] Some of the most popular users tried to turn their followings into financially profitable endeavors, but the leftist/anti-capitalist politics of these users made their economic aspirations more about supporting themselves and being able to make a living than directly selling products to their followers in the vein that social media influencers tend to do.

One such user posts under the handle @binchcity, but also displays her real name, Julia Hava, on her profile. She had 49,100 followers in late 2018, and at the time of writing in June 2022, she has 123,000 followers. In the bio-section of Hava's Instagram profile, there is a link to her personal website where one can purchase her memes as posters, t-shirts, stickers, or mugs.[93] Hava also has a Patreon site, where one can support her work monthly.[94] Patreon is a platform which allows content creators to set up multitiered subscription programs for their fans, where followers pay a fixed amount each month to get access to premium content and support the work of the creator. This form of financing has become very popular among digital creators, with several creative workers living off their Patreon subscriptions.[95] For the sad girls on Instagram, to have a Patreon as well as selling merchandise, like Hava does, becomes a way to turn the large followings they have into actual financial rewards, without going through the sponsorship deals that are common among more mainstream influencers. But it is important to note that this does not necessarily mean that their followers do contribute in any large numbers or at all, when they can get most of the content for free on Instagram.

Hava's memes often take the shape of commercial illustrations that look like they might be from the 1950s or 1960s overlaid with her own comedic words. One example is an image of a woman in a flowing dress holding a medication bottle (that looks like it has been photoshopped into her hand) next to the words "Girls just wanna have SEROTONIN"[96] (see Fig. 5.5). Hava has captioned the image "remember to smash your mf [motherfucking] medication today everyone" and at the time of writing it

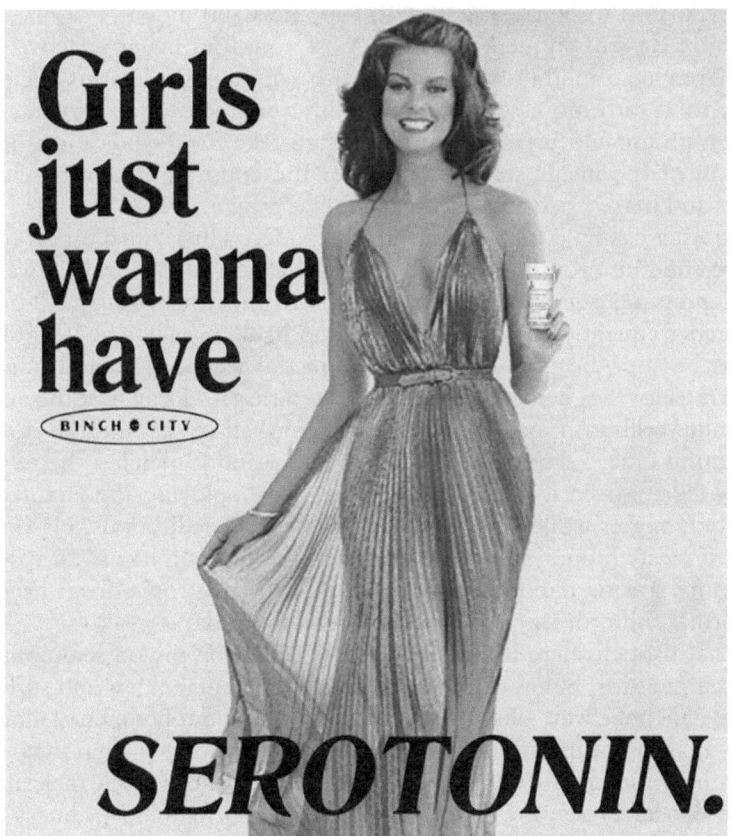

Fig. 5.5 "Girls just wanna have Serotonin," meme by Julia Hava, @binchcity

has 20,399 likes and 475 comments. In relation to Blackman's notion of suffering as ordinary, posts like these serve the same function as the above-mentioned examples from Tumblr that connects summer vacation with isolation and severe depression.[97] In the case of Hava's Instagram posts, what is implied is not (only) a base level of constant sadness but that her followers are all taking some kind of prescription drug for depression. The phrase "Girls just wanna have SEROTONIN" is a play on several things: the 1983 hit song by Cyndi Lauper, the 1985 romantic comedy film, and the more recent signage "Girls just wanna have fundamental rights," part of popular feminist branding and available for purchase on t-shirt, mugs, stickers, and posters on sites like Etsy. The neurotransmitter serotonin is widely known to be associated with happiness and mood, with the most common class of antidepressants in most countries being selective serotonin reuptake inhibitors (SSRIs) which (in simplified terms) help the brain to absorb more serotonin.[98] By inserting serotonin into the well-known phrase and urging her followers to take their medications in the caption of the image, Hava normalizes the consumption of psychiatric drugs and makes it part of everyday life.

Another example from Hava is a short video of her "medication haul," where she humorously shows off her medication holder and the various antidepressants she is taking, in the style of the "makeup hauls" beauty vloggers frequently engage in. A "makeup haul" usually involves a show-and-tell of new beauty products,[99] and in this video, Hava addresses her viewers as lovelies before showing off two different dosages of the antidepressant Wellbutrin, one in a "beautiful eggshell color" and the other in "beautiful blue, I would say kinda baby blue and it matches the medication holder, so perfect coordination."[100] By employing the language of beauty bloggers while describing her psychiatric medications, Hava manages to create humor and irony around both "makeup hauls" and antidepressants. Taking antidepressants and other psychotropic drugs becomes as normal and ordinary as wearing makeup every day.

What happens here is similar to the normalizing discourse among the Tumblr sad girls, but as opposed to glorifying mental illness and suffering in a melancholic way, what Hava does is to joke about her mental illness in a way that can be interpreted as crass and self-defeating (within the humor styles mentioned above).[101] Here again is an example of normalization's ambivalence. Presenting psychiatric drugs as normal and ordinary does not necessarily challenge any systems or question definitions of what it means to be mentally ill or healthy. In a way the distanced approach to her own struggles taken by Hava can be read as similar to *Cosmopolitan's* tongue-in-cheek writing about mental health and as a clear example of the relatability Kanai describes in women's media culture and that involves a display yet disavowal of injury.

Within this framework, Hava and the other Instagram sad girls who post similar content may be deemed to make light of serious health issues by turning them into self-defeating comedy. But seen instead in a context where psychiatric diagnoses are something to be ashamed of, the open display of one's diagnoses and medications becomes an act of defiance against normative discourses. The humor employed here can then be read more as "affiliative" in the sense that it is shared in a social media network with the purpose of connecting to others who have similar experiences of living with mental illness.[102] The use of humor here may be read as diminishing the seriousness of mental illness, but it also becomes a way for sufferers to connect to each other and (possibly) feel less alone. And crucially, the display of vulnerability here is not of the kind common in confidence culture——where difficulties are shared after they have been successfully overcome——but rather a display of the real-time experience of taking a range of psychiatric medications as part of everyday life. Hava's medication haul then is not an example of profitable vulnerability, but rather of a capacious sad girl culture where humor is employed to make fun of both the practice of keeping track of multiple medications and the consumer logic behind makeup haul videos.

Another popular user is Ghosted1996 who only displays her first name Haley on her profile.[103] Haley lives with bipolar disorder and frequently posts about that and the medications she takes. The comedic aspect of the memes is often accompanied by a critique of capitalism and the health care system in the U.S. For example, one of Haley's early posts is a mockup of an advertisement for the antipsychotic drug Seroquel which is often used in the treatment of bipolar disorder.[104] A picture of a woman with wavy hair is laid on top of the Seroquel name and logo and a blurry version of the side effects text that usually accompanies medication advertisements, and Haley's own words spell out:

> People always ask me how I attain my flawless beach waves. I tell them, 'Well, my medication gives me night sweats/terrors and I wake up drenched every morning along with numerous other side effects (some dangerous) that are irrelevant to the pharmaceutical industry because they care more about profit than healthcare.'[105] (See Fig. 5.6)

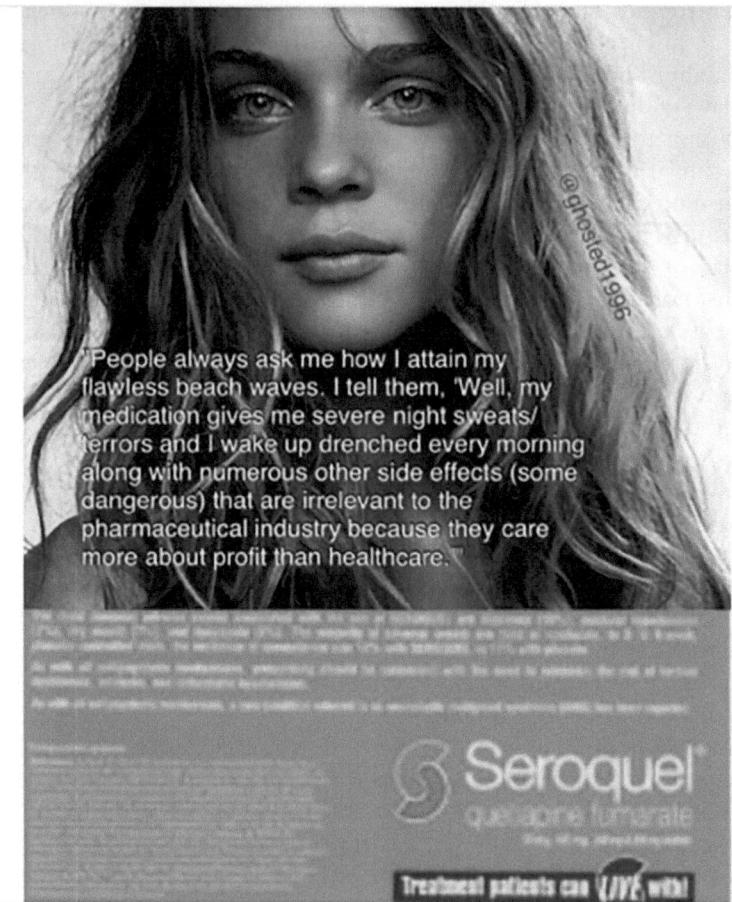

Fig. 5.6 Seroquel meme by Haley Byam, @ghosted1996

In the comments section Haley's followers express the resonance of the post with one user saying "hahahahhahaahaha why is this me exactly wow haha seroquel amiright" and others talking about how various drugs have given them night sweats and other side effects. Another example is a meme with two images of actor Shia LaBeouf looking distraught and Haley's text reading:

Me looking at the state of mental health care in this country and wondering how the fuck mentally ill ppl are expected to go through the arduous process of applying and being accepted for disability benefits if their own doctors (let alone the state or federal government) refuse to take them seriously.[106] (Fig. 5.7)

In the comments section people are posting emojis high-five:ing and sharing their own stories of being diagnosed and misdiagnosed and prescribed various medications, and of having to pay large amounts of money to stay insured or simply not having access to care.

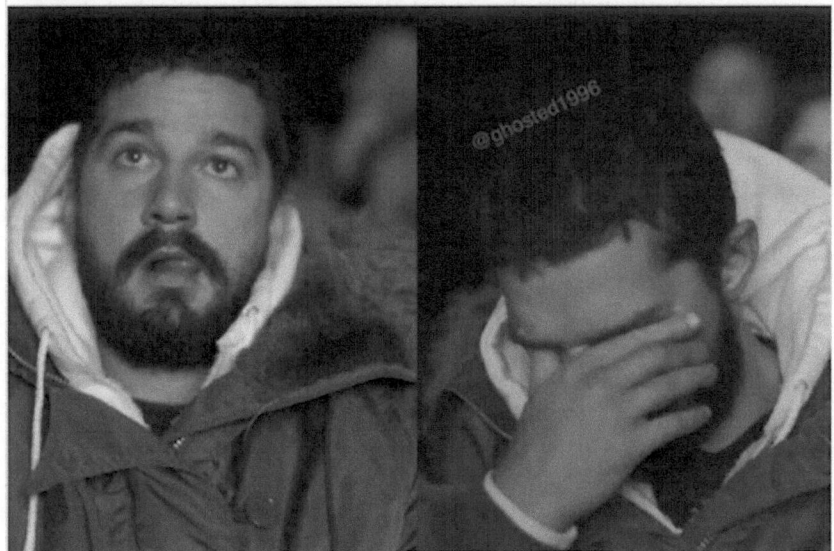

Fig. 5.7 Meme about the US healthcare system by Haley Byam, @ghosted1996

Again, within the various humor styles outlined above, the comedic style of Hava and Haley might be read as aggressive or self-defeating, and thus more likely to belong to someone with a depression diagnosis and can possibly lead to negative effects on health.[107] Some of the humor displayed by Haley can be read as self-effacing and harsh, but the engagement with both of the above posts show how such dark comedy also can function as a node around which Instagram users can gather and provide support to each other. This shows the potential of this platform and the internet in general to function as a supportive space for individuals suffering from mental distress. Through the medium of humorous memes, people share their despair and frustrations and can be made to feel less alone. Haley herself said so directly when she was interviewed by Paper Magazine in January 2019 after having been named one of "100 People Taking Over 2019" by the outlet. In the interview she spoke about the support she has gotten from the Instagram community, saying:

> I've been running my account for about two years now, and the unprecedented amount of healing I've found in the meme community feels like the answer to a question I've never been able to articulate. I'm truly grateful to be a part of this space in time, where conceivably anyone can access free content that assures them they're not alone or crazy for struggling. For a long time I felt like everything I went through was meaningless, but connecting with people who understand me and actually feel comforted by the things I make has shown me I'm capable of creating a silver lining.[108]

This shows the supportive potential of these online spaces. The role of humor here is similar to what has been described by feminist media studies scholars in relation to feminist online discourses that employ comedy for community building and consciousness raising.[109] In the discussion of the Twitter account @NoToFeminism, which uses humor to rebuke anti-feminist discourse online, Emilie Lawrence and Jessica Ringrose write that "the account draws attention to instances of systematic inequality and injustice through humor rather than anger, frustration, or the sadness characteristic of being a 'victim' of sexism."[110] The result is that followers and participants are offered "new, potentially empowering, ways to understand and engage with topics like the wage gap and sexual violence," something that Lawrence and Ringrose mark as "potentially therapeutic."[111] I think a similar thing can be said about the comedic tone among the sad girls on Instagram and how the humor becomes a way to distance oneself from the difficulties of living with mental illness and at the same time feel less alone.

Another aspect of the shared comedic discourse created here is the literacy that is required to understand and "get" the jokes being shared. Kanai analyzes this in relation to the Tumblr-blog WhatShouldWeCallMe and the memes that circulated among the original creators and its follower blogs. She argues that there is a specific set of "conceptual and socially predicated readerly knowledges [that] enable the literacy required for participation" in this meme.[112] In Kanai's example the memes are closely tied to "contemporary feminine practices and digital cultures" and imply an immersion in these discourses.[113] In the context of the Instagram sad girls the shared literacy instead concerns having personal experiences of mental illness and psychiatric medications, and in the case of the examples from Haley mentioned above, a firsthand knowledge of the US mental health care system.

Possibilities of Sadness and Political Potential

Another aspect that complicates the relatability of the Instagram sad girls and which is very much part of their shared literacy is the explicit political engagement among them. Whereas the Tumblr sad girls can be read as exploring the potential of impasse and resting in sadness by refusing to work immediately toward a cure, their counterparts on Instagram are often explicitly political. An example in addition to Haley's memes about the US health care system mentioned above is a post by user manicpixie-memequeen. This meme features a photo of a woman lying down on a bench at the mall, staring sadly into her phone and holding several shopping bags. On top of the image a text reads: "walking around the mall realizing that we are all slaves to the inescapable system of capitalism that benefits from the exploitation of our labor & our insatiable meaningless desires" and as a caption manicpixiememequeen has written simply "sad socialist memes."[114] (Fig. 5.8). Another example of this outright political analysis found among the sad girls on Instagram is a post by user @prozac. barbie that features a photo of Kendall Jenner looking sad accompanied by the text "real photo of me trying to reconcile my hatred of the capitalist society I'm part of with my insatiable appetite for material objects I falsely believe will bring me the happiness I crave."[115] By inserting political analysis into the stream of sad girl content on the platform, followers learn to associate also critical, anti-capitalist, thought into the experience of mental illness, and connections can possibly be made between personal suffering and larger, structural issues. The posts here could also be read as

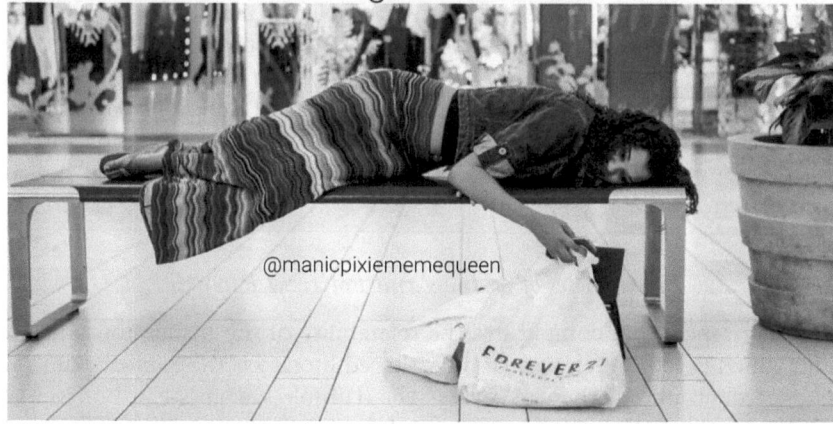

Fig. 5.8 "Walking around the mall/Sad socialist memes" by @ manicpixiememequeen

presenting an alternative to commercialized self-care discourses that encourage consumption to soothe one's anxieties.

This also speaks to the shared literacy assumed in these online spaces. In addition to knowing what it is like to live with various mental health issues, the reader of these memes is also assumed to understand and agree with an anti-capitalist worldview that holds the above analyses of the consumption culture and its role in society. This is similar to the "insider/outsider dynamics of being part of a clever, intersectional feminist sensibility" that Lawrence and Ringrose describe in feminist discourses on Twitter.[116] Here the humorous tweets "encourage critical thinking by inviting audiences to be part of a complex set of understandings about power and privilege" that is part of this "intersectional feminist sensibility."[117] A similar sensibility is being encouraged among the sad girls on Instagram, but in relation to mental health and capitalism instead of intersectional feminism (although these themes are also present among these sad girls).

Sad Girls Club

Sad Girls Club is an Instagram account that focuses specifically on providing support and quickly gained traction on the platform. It was started in February 2017 by the filmmaker Elyse Fox, who after releasing a short film about her own struggles with depression (titled *Conversations With Friends*) heard from girls from all over the world who thanked her for telling her story.[118] Judging from the activity on her Instagram profile, Fox did not have a large following before starting Sad Girls Club, but gained micro-celebrity status after the club became popular on the platform (at the time of writing she has 37,000 followers on her private account and the club has 261,000 followers). Looking back at her posts there was an increase in the average number of likes and comments on her posts after Instagram featured Fox and Sad Girls Club on their official account to mark the mental health awareness campaign #HereForYou that the platform organized in May 2017.[119]

The club itself, frequently with Fox as a spokesperson, received a lot of coverage in various media outlets, including mainstream publications like *Forbes, SELF* magazine, *Women's Health,* and NBC's the TODAY show blog.[120] This suggests that a narrative of helping young women battle mental illness was something that was given attention in the mainstream media at the time, and that aligning yourself with mental health awareness causes was a good branding strategy. The logic in much of this mainstream coverage resembles the language of mental health advocacy employed primarily by *Teen Vogue*. For example, the headline of the *SELF* magazine story about Sad Girls Club reads "How Instagram's 'Sad Girls Club' Is Busting the Stigma Around Mental Illness," which aligns with the awareness discourse that emphasizes the importance of speaking out as discussed in Chap. 3.[121] Representatives from Sad Girls Club also attended the 2018 *Teen Vogue* summit, showing the connections between the magazine and this part of Instagram sad girl discourse.[122] Fox also participated in marketing campaigns for the beauty brand Olay and the fashion brand Monki, where she was presented as a mental health advocate, showing the commercial viability of mental health awareness at this point in time.[123]

In contrast to the accounts mentioned above, Sad Girls Club did not only post memes for other users to recognize themselves in, but had a clear community focus and arranged in-person meetings in New York City, where those in need of support could come together to provide it for each other. Fox, who is African-American, also emphasized that she wanted to support women of color specifically in their struggle with mental illness. In an interview with *SELF* magazine, she said that the tools to treat and cope with mental illnesses are widely available, but what is missing is a fair representation of who struggles with it. What is missing is "a woman of color who's saying, 'I have a mental illness and I'm happy; I'm living my life and this is how I do it.'"[124] This is important in relation to the above-mentioned tensions between the various definitions of the sad girl and the stereotypical sad girl as someone who has relied primarily on "white bodies as a way of presenting depressive themes and exploring girlhood."[125] What Fox has done with the Sad Girls Club is to adopt the term sad girl as one that encompasses multiple racial identities. By speaking about the lack of nonwhite representations of mental illness she opens up the figure for identification by girls and others from a range of subject positions, not only white can-do girls who are fed up with the demands of white girlhood, but also girls of color whose struggles might have to do with issues like systemic racism and disenfranchisement.

Sad Girls Club typically posts content that focuses mostly on providing support, like an infographic about how to help a friend with depression or a multi-image post about the importance of fighting the stigma surrounding mental health.[126] When thinking about Blackman's notion of suffering as ordinary, the activity of the Sad Girls Club could be seen as fulfilling this notion by merely normalizing psychic suffering and advocating for the acknowledgment of mental health issues as an everyday part of life that affects a significant amount of people.[127] But whereas the sad girls on Tumblr tend to rest in a melancholic stance that glorifies feeling bad, and the other sad girls on Instagram rely on humor and comedy to come together around shared difficulties, Sad Girls Club puts the focus on support. This is not to say that the other kinds of sad girls do not provide support, or that Sad Girls Club never posts humorous posts. The club often posts memes, but the overall emphasis is on providing support to other Instagram users and to create space where users can express themselves and share their feelings, seen in prompts to engage with each other in the comments sections. One example of this is a post about what to do if you have a friend that is sharing things online that makes you worried about their mental health.[128] Here Sad Girls Club is sharing a humorous meme about posting negative things, but by asking what their followers do in the kind of situation described they are opening up for a more serious reading of what might be going on behind the comedic and relatable facade. And most importantly, they are encouraging their followers to connect with each other, which in itself can relieve symptoms by making those who suffer feel less alone.

My Therapist Says: The Acritical and Commercialized Sad Girl Aesthetic

It is also worth mentioning the Instagram account @mytherapistsays, as an example of profitable vulnerability in the worlds of social media. The account was started in 2015 and reached over two million followers in its first two years (at the time of writing it has 7.5 million followers).[129] It was founded by best friends Lola Tash and Nicole Argiris, who lived in separate cities and decided to start a shared account to post memes. By virtue of its name, the account purports to deal with mental health, but the content frequently covered a more generalized worry regarding "their anxiety-prone twentysomething lives: aggressive crush texting, impulsive shopping, canceling plans in order to sleep."[130] On the spectrum of peer support, micro-celebrity, and influencers, My Therapist Says represents the most acritical and commercialized version of the mental illness discourse happening on these platforms. The two women behind the account have managed to monetize it by turning it into a multifaceted social media brand, complete with an accompanying blog, merchandise shop, and book.

My Therapist Says rarely went into detail about medications or diagnoses, like the users mentioned above (ghosted1996, binchcity, etc.), and the critical messages found among the Instagram sad girls were completely absent. Instead the women running the account collaborated with big brands like (makeup company) Urban Decay and (dating app) Tinder to produce sponsored content to share with their followers.[131] In early 2020 @mytherapistsays was also one of the Instagram accounts involved in presidential candidate Michael Bloomberg's campaign's push to reach out to voters via memes.[132] This indicates the clout and presumed influence that the account posits also among the mainstream meme-creators on the platform.

My Therapist Says is very similar to the Tumblr-blog WhatShouldWeCallMe that Kanai studies, down to the fact that both were started by friends living geographically apart who started a public documentation of their friendship in the form of memes.[133] The same mechanisms of converting frustrations into "funny, bitesized moments" which "produce selves amenable to circulation in a gendered, digital economy of relatability" are at play in both WhatShouldWeCallMe and My Therapist Says.[134] The latter frequently manages to take anxieties about working, socializing and having a larger "put together" life and turn them into easily digestible memes. One example that plays on several layers of intertextuality is a photograph of Britney Spears riding in a miniature car made for children (made apparent by the fact that she is much too big for it) accompanied by the text "when u try to act like u got ur life together but clearly shit is falling apart."[135] In the caption Tash and Argiris have written "Forever always on the verge of a Britney 2007 meltdown," a reference to the public breakdown that the singer went through which was framed as a "trainwreck" (as I discussed in Chap. 4) and has spawned a large number of Internet commentary and memes.[136] The follower who sees this post will presumably recognize themselves in the feeling of things falling apart, but then that potentially threatening feeling is defused by the humorous image of Spears in the miniature car, and the person viewing the image is presumably left just calmed enough to be able to participate in daily life again.

My Therapist Says also follows Gill and Kanai's analysis of the "feeling rules" of neoliberalism and the display yet disavowal of injuries common in contemporary media culture, in the way difficult subjects are taken up but only to be immediately made fun of.[137] The fact that Tash and Argiris have successfully turned their Instagram account into a profitable social media company underscores the value of the "gendered, digital economy of relatability."[138] The focus on relatability was even laid out in the official brand mission of My Therapist Says, which was displayed in their media kit and in the advertising section of their website which at one point read "the goal of MyTherapistSays was to be a relatable brand, speaking to struggles of a 20 to 30 something woman who's a bit of a mess."[139]

The account is an example of turning one's followers' worries and anxieties into literal financial rewards, in the sense that it is through their highly relatable content about everyday anxieties that Tash and Argiris have built their following, and it is due to their high number of followers that they can charge companies for advertisements and sponsored content. The two women have managed to toe the line of expressing frustrations with contemporary life without sounding like too much or becoming threatening, while also excelling at entrepreneurial adaptability in realizing early on that they could monetize their relatability. My Therapist Says is thus a clear example of the profitability of certain kinds of vulnerability.

A PRECARITY-FOCUSED CONSCIOUSNESS RAISING

I want to propose that some of the sad girls discussed above are examples of the kind of "precarity-focused consciousness raising" suggested by the *Institute for Precarious Consciousness*. This scholarly activist collective argues in their 2014 manifesto "We are all very anxious" that anxiety is the dominant affect that holds contemporary capitalism together, and that it functions to control and maintain the unequal status quo. For them this anxiety is closely connected to precarity and the precarious living conditions of contemporary capitalism. One defining aspect of the dominant affect is that it is a public secret, "something that everyone knows, but nobody admits, or talks about."[140] The secrecy is a powerful tool in keeping the affect in place as it keeps it personalized and blame or cause for the anxiety is placed on the individual rather than the larger social and cultural structures which shape the individual's living conditions. But the *Institute* argues that the dominant affect can be broken down by exposing its social sources, and they advocate a "style of precarity-focused consciousness raising" to move out from under the debilitating grip of anxiety. Taking inspiration from feminist consciousness raising of the 1960s and 1970s, the collective proposes a form of political action that involves "analysing and theorising structural sources based on similarities in experience."[141] I contend that the sad girls on Tumblr and Instagram are practicing a version of such a consciousness raising.

The *Institute* presents six points of focus for such a practice. First, precarity-focused consciousness raising must be "Producing new grounded theory relating to experience," meaning that political theory and activist practice needs to connect with the experiences of living in the present rather than older models for understanding power and oppression. The *Institute* writes, "the idea here is that our own perceptions of our situation are blocked or cramped by dominant assumptions, and need to be made explicit." Secondly, a precarity-focused consciousness raising must "[Recognise] the reality, and the systemic nature, of our experiences," which involves affirming "that our pain is really pain, that what we see and feel is real, and that our problems are not only personal".[142] Both of these points are seen in the Instagram posts about the defunct mental health care system in the U.S. and the profit incentives of big pharmaceutical companies mentioned above, and the conversations that happen in the comments section of these posts where other Instagram users share their own experiences of navigating the health care system and trying different medications.[143] Another example is a post, also from Haley (@ ghosted1996), featuring a picture of Uma Thurman in the movie *Kill Bill*, holding up a sword that she seems ready to slay someone with. Above the image Haley has written "me every time I try a new hormonal birth control, knowing that my entire life could be destroyed in the ensuing months while all the cis men around me carry none of this responsibility or risk" while the caption reads: "Anyone tried nuva ring for PMDD? Drop ur experiences in the comments below."[144] Among the 193 comments people share their experiences of trying various birth control, and together with Haley's original post, this becomes a small forum where a knowledge of what it means to live through these things is formed and shared.

The third point mentioned by the *Institute* is that a precarity-focused consciousness raising must involve a "Transformation of emotions," which they explain by saying that "people are paralysed by unnameable emotions, and a general sense of feeling like shit" and clarifying that "these emotions need to be transformed into a sense of injustice, a type of anger which is less resentful and more focused, a move towards self-expression, and a reactivation of resistance."[145] There is a transformation of emotions happening among the sad girls on both Tumblr and Instagram, but most of the emotions get transformed into humor and a sense of "not being alone," so there are ways to go before turning them into an anger that drives action, which the *Institute* advocates for.

Fourth on the list of what a precarity-focused consciousness raising should entail is "Creating or expressing voice," expanded on as "the culture of silence surrounding the public secret needs to be overthrown."[146] This requirement is met by the sad girls by virtue of the public display of their sadness and other mental illnesses, and the shared voice that is formed within that discourse. The next point on the *Institute's* list is the "[Construction of] a disalienated space," which would serve as a sort of safe space to provide "critical distance on one's life, and a kind of emotional safety net to attempt transformations, dissolving fears." The manifesto clarifies that "this should not simply be a self-help measure, used to sustain existing activities, but instead, a space for reconstructing a radical perspective." The more outright supportive accounts in the online sad girl discourse, like Sad Girls Club, are examples of this kind of disalienated space. Although these spaces are more about providing direct support and relief, there may be a few steps left before the radical perspective proposed by the *Institute* is fully realized. The last point/issue that the *Institute* lists as crucial for a precarity-focused consciousness raising is "Analysing and theorising structural sources based on similarities in experience," expanded on as "the point is not simply to recount experiences but to transform and restructure them through their theorisation." So this would be the practice of using the knowledge gained through a multitude of individual experiences to form a theory of how structures of power and resources work. Wollen's Sad Girl Theory and the art she shared via her Instagram account and in interviews are examples of practices that seem to fit with this point, in the act of politicizing sadness as a protest against patriarchal culture. The disappearance of Wollen from the platform and her subsequent deletion of the sad girl content speaks to the limitations of using a corporate platform like Instagram for radical political projects. Haley's (@ghosted1996) Instagram account was also removed from the platform in late 2021, due to an unclear violation of community guidelines (but she is still active on the platform under the slightly different username @ghosted_1996).[147] Instances like this show the precariousness of relying on private platforms whose enactment of rules is often shrouded in an air of secrecy.

CONCLUSION

In this chapter I have discussed various ways in which young women have written about their sadness on social media, primarily under the sad girl moniker. For some sad girl figures (My Therapist Says), the feeling-rules of neoliberalism are promoted. Others (Tumblr and Instagram sad girls, Wollen, and Sad Girls Y Qué) contest them explicitly while others (Sad Girls Club) are seeking precarious forms of solidarity.

Relatability is present in various ways in all of the examples of sad girls discussed in this chapter, where the display of vulnerability is often accompanied by something humorous so as to make it less serious. But this relatability is employed in different ways by the different actors involved. My Therapist Says creates memes about smaller anxieties to sustain their brand of relatability in a more lighthearted way that makes them appealing enough for partnerships with big companies like Tinder and Urban Decay. The sad girls on Instagram——like Hava, Haley, and @manicpixiememequeen——create memes about heavier topics that are relatable to those who share their experiences of various diagnoses but also their opinions on the US health care system and late-stage capitalism. In this figuration the humor does not turn the experiences into "funny, bitesized moments" that fit into "a gendered, digital economy of relatability,"[148] but functions as a coping mechanism that creates connections between the sad girls and their followers, who can come together in their despair over the state of the world and their psyches. A similar thing happened among the sad girls on Tumblr, in their practice of resting in sadness and the exploration of the impasse of acedia and melancholia found there. Like this the sad girls of Tumblr and Instagram represent a kind of rupture in the relatability paradigm, in that those participating in these discourses are encouraged to consider depression, anxiety, and mental illness as central aspects of life rather than something to immediately laugh off. This is also why they can represent a way forward for the kind of precarity-focused consciousness raising that the *Institute for Precarious Consciousness* proposes.

Regardless of the platforms, there is a key tension that runs through sad girl aesthetics and communities: there is a risk here of glorifying sadness and mental illness, but paradoxically in the very act of sharing one's feelings online one also learns that one is not alone. In this way all of the examples discussed here do provide some level of support to their followers. In some cases, providing support is an explicit mission and cause, like for the Sad Girls Club. While in others it is an indirect effect of a comedic and sometimes irreverent discourse where followers might come to the profiles of the Instagram sad girls for the memes and to laugh at things that are otherwise serious, but then indirectly they find support in discovering that others feel the same way they do.

By forming discourses where multiple voices and experiences of living with mental illness get to be heard, alternative and multifaceted ways of conceptualizing sadness become available in these online spaces. This gives sufferers access to a potentially supportive collective of other sufferers. Here, those who fail to be helped by traditional psychiatric discourse can get a chance to be heard, learn that they are not alone, and possibly receive non-medicalized modes of support.

NOTES

1. Hines, "a taxonomy of the sad girl."
2. Newell-Hanson, "2015 the year of... sad girls and sad boys."
3. Alderton, *The aesthetics of self-harm*, xx.
4. Devcollab, "The Reign Of The Internet Sad Girl Is Over;" Joho, "How being sad, depressed, and anxious online became trendy;" Mondalek, "When did it become cool to be a 'sad girl'?;" Petrarca, "A Memes to an End;" Saxelby, "Meet Bunny Michael, The Artist Whose Tragicomic Memes Say What Everyone Is Feeling."

5. Barron, "richard prince, audrey wollen, and the sad girl theory;" Tunnicliffe, "Audrey Wollen On The Power of Sadness;" Watson, "How girls are finding empowerment through being sad online;" Wells, "Audrey Wollen's Feminist Instagram World."
6. Montgomery, "@SoSadToday: Twitter's Favorite Depressive Breaks Her Silence;" Vozick-Levinson, "@SoSadToday Reveals Herself."
7. Decaille, "Elyse Fox's "Sad Girls Club" Challenges The Narrative About Women Of Color & Mental Health;" Fluker, "How Founder Of Sad Girls Club Tackles Mental Health Issues Online;" Jacoby, "How Instagram's 'Sad Girls Club' Is Busting the Stigma Around Mental Illness;" Ross, "Elyse Fox: 'I Was Labeled As The Angry Black Woman.'"
8. Jennings, "Wearing Your Emotions on Your Sleeve;" Pandika, "Sad culture normalizes mental illness."
9. Duggan et al, "An Examination of the Scope and Nature of Non-Suicidal Self-Injury Online Activities;" Jadayel, Medlej, and Jadayel, "Mental Disorders: a Glamorous Attraction on Social Media?;" Seko et al, "On the creative edge: Exploring motivations for creating non-suicidal self-injury content online;" Whitlock, Powers, and Eckenrode, "The virtual cutting edge: The Internet and adolescent self-injury."
10. McCosker, "Engaging mental health online;" Tucker and Goodings, "Medicated bodies: Mental distress, social media and affect."
11. Holowka, "Between artifice and emotion: the "sad girls" of Instagram;" Mooney, "Sad Girls and Carefree Black Girls;" My own piece about Tumblr sad girls was published in *Capacious: Journal for Emerging Affect Inquiry* in 2017, and part of what I discussed there is repeated here, and can thus be seen to have contributed to the scholarly conversation about sad girls as well, Thelandersson, "Social Media Sad Girls and the Normalization of Sad States of Being."
12. Gray, "The Question of Cultural Appropriation."
13. Alderton, *The aesthetics of self-harm*, 95.
14. Ibid, 95.
15. Ibid, 95, italicization in original.
16. Kanai, "Sociality and Classification: Reading Gender, Race, and Class in a Humorous Meme."
17. Gill and Kanai, "Mediating Neoliberal Capitalism;" Hochschild, *The Managed Heart.*
18. Gill and Kanai, "Mediating Neoliberal Capitalism," 323.
19. Orgad and Gill, *Confidence Culture.*
20. Ibid, 96.
21. Gibbs, "Apparently unrelated: Affective resonance, concatenation and traumatic circuitry in the terrain of the everyday," 131-132.
22. Ibid, 133.

23. Bratich, "Occupy All the Dispositifs," 2.
24. Ibid, 3.
25. Alfonso, "The real origins of Tumblr."
26. Premack, "Tumblr's Depression Connection."
27. Cho, "Default publicness: Queer youth of color, social media, and being outed by the machine;" Fink and Miller, "Trans media moments: Tumblr, 2011-2013;" Morimoto and Stein, "Tumblr and fandom."
28. Renninger, "'Where I can be myself… where I can speak my mind,'" 5.
29. In a 2018 study of the most popular social media platforms among college students Tumblr did not make the cut as one of the top sites, as not enough participants named it as their favorite platform. Shane-Simpson et al, "Why do college students prefer Facebook, Twitter, or Instagram?," 279.
30. Grvnge-nicotine, "Medicated," Tumblr post, accessed June 22, 2022, https://grvnge-nicotine.tumblr.com/post/115523875193/grunge-baby; Less-love-more-alcohol, "100% Sad," Tumblr post, accessed June 22, 2022, http://less-love-more-alcohol.tumblr.com/post/158888514189/successfulling; Animatedtext, "Having a threesome with anxiety and depression," Tumblr post, accessed June 22, 2022, https://animatedtext.tumblr.com/post/142548878872/requested-by-0n-your-knees; Hollywood-noir, "Lisa Simpson Sad Girl," Tumblr post, accessed June 22, 2022, https://hollywood-noir.tumblr.com/post/116832925747/soft-grunge.
31. Havic-dp, "Pills," Tumblr post, accessed June 22, 2022, https://havic-dp.tumblr.com/post/90219378205.
32. Sweet-despondency, "I told my therapist about you," Tumblr post, accessed June 22, 2022, https://sweet-despondency.tumblr.com/post/148574795828.
33. Alderton, *The aesthetics of self-harm*; Renninger, "'Where I can be myself… where I can speak my mind.'"
34. See http://grvnge-nicotine.tumblr.com and http://hollywood-noir.tumblr.com, both accessed June 22, 2022.
35. Blackman, "Affective politics, debility and hearing voices," 26. See also Blackman, *Hearing Voices*; Blackman and Walkerdine, *Mass hysteria*.
36. Blackman, "Affective politics, debility and hearing voices," 26.
37. Ibid, 26.
38. Straightboyfriend, "its summer vacation you know what that means!," Tumblr post, accessed June 22, 2022, https://straightboyfriend.tumblr.com/post/145484278234/its-summer-vacation-you-know-what-that-means.
39. Gothicprep, "how do i contour my abandonment issues?," Tumblr post, accessed June 22, 2022, https://gothicprep.tumblr.com/post/139090742155/how-do-i-contour-my-abandonment-issues.

40. Freud, "Humour," 216. See also Freud, *Jokes and Their Relation to the Unconscious.*
41. O'Connell, "Freudian humour," 327.
42. Martin and Lefcourt, "Sense of humor as a moderator of the relation between stressors and moods," 1314.
43. Ibid, 1322.
44. Martin et al, "Individual differences in uses of humor and their relation to psychological well-being."
45. Greengross, "The Relationship Between Humor and Depression."
46. Martin et al, "Individual differences in uses of humor and their relation to psychological well-being," 48.
47. Greengross, "The Relationship Between Humor and Depression."
48. Kfrerer, Martin and Schermer, "A behavior genetic analysis of the relationship between humor styles and depression."
49. Kanai, "Sociality and Classification: Reading Gender, Race, and Class in a Humorous Meme."
50. Rentschler and Thrift, "Doing feminism in the network," 329; see also Lawrence and Ringrose, "@Notofeminism, #Feministsareugly, and Misandry Memes."
51. Blackman, "Affective politics, debility and hearing voices," 25.
52. Cvetkovich, *Depression: A public feeling,* 21.
53. Ibid, 21.
54. Blackman, "Affective politics, debility and hearing voices."
55. Hollywood-noir, "Self-destructive and unproductive," Tumblr post, accessed June 22, 2022, https://hollywood-noir.tumblr.com/post/141516412702; Paintdeath, "I've Been Crying All Day," Tumblr post, accessed June 22, 2022, https://paintdeath.tumblr.com/post/146787727149/cant-wait-to-wear-this-everyday; Fattyacidtrip, "Trying to write my resume like...," Tumblr post, accessed June 22, 2022, https://fattyacidtrip.tumblr.com/post/103235397341.
56. Cvetkovich, *Depression: A public feeling,* 85.
57. Ibid, 102.
58. Ibid, 107.
59. Berlant, *Desire/Love,* 29.
60. m1nd--0ver—matter, "You like your girls insane," Tumblr post, accessed June 22, 2022, https://m1nd%2D%2D0ver%2D%2Dmatter.tumblr.com/post/120501681047.
61. Got-You-Where-I-Want-You, Tumblr post, accessed June 22, 2022, http://got-you-where-i-want-you.tumblr.com/post/158824899040; Sweet-Despondency, Tumblr post, accessed June 22, 2022, https://sweet-despondency.tumblr.com/post/147347687983/mothurs-candid-photo-of-lucifer-and-the-angel.

62. Hollywood-noir, "sext: I want to be good for your mental health," Tumblr post, accessed June 22, 2022, http://hollywood-noir.tumblr.com/post/125186281077/flowers-in-my-hair-demons-in-my-head.
63. Holowka, "Between artifice and emotion: the "sad girls" of Instagram."
64. Gonzalez and Wollen, "In Conversation with Mira Gonzalez;" Watson, "How girls are finding empowerment through being sad online."
65. Wells, "Audrey Wollen's Feminist Instagram World."
66. Wollen in Tunnicliffe, "Audrey Wollen On The Power of Sadness."
67. Wollen in Barron, "richard prince, audrey wollen, and the sad girl theory."
68. Ibid.
69. Gill and Kanai, "Mediating Neoliberal Capitalism;" Gill and Orgad, "The Confidence Cult(ure);" Orgad and Gill, *Confidence Culture*.
70. Barron, "richard prince, audrey wollen, and the sad girl theory;" Tunnicliffe, "Audrey Wollen On The Power of Sadness;" Watson, "How girls are finding empowerment through being sad online;" Wells, "Audrey Wollen's Feminist Instagram World."
71. Wells, "Audrey Wollen's Feminist Instagram World."
72. Barron, "richard prince, audrey wollen, and the sad girl theory."
73. Alderton, *The aesthetics of self-harm*, 100.
74. Marwick, "Instafame: Luxury selfies in the attention economy," 334.
75. Ibid.
76. Wollen in Eler, "Panel This is What Feminism 4.0 Looks Like."
77. Ibid.
78. Jones, "Remembering Instagram Before the Influencers."
79. Ibid.
80. Calderón-Douglass, "Sad Girls y Qué Are Breaking Down Machismo with Internet Art;" Eden, "Sad Girls Y Qué."
81. The group also had a Twitter account, and at the time of writing both this and the Facebook page are still available, but they have not been active since April 2016.
82. Calderón-Douglass, "Sad Girls y Qué Are Breaking Down Machismo with Internet Art."
83. Urban Dictionary, "Sad Girl," website entry, September 7, 2006, accessed June 25, 2022, https://www.urbandictionary.com/define.php?term=Sad%20Girl.
84. Calderón-Douglass, "Sad Girls y Qué Are Breaking Down Machismo with Internet Art."
85. Alderton, *The aesthetics of self-harm*, 106.
86. Lana del Rey, "Tropico (Short Film)," Youtube video, December 6, 2013, accessed June 25, 2022, https://www.youtube.com/watch?v=VwuHOQLSpEg.
87. Mooney, "Sad Girls and Carefree Black Girls," 184.

88. Ibid, 184, 190.
89. Ibid, 190.
90. In 2019 Instagram started experimenting with removing the total number of likes from a post, for a while users in several countries could no longer display how many likes singular posts received. At the time of writing, however, users can choose to either show or hide the exact number of likes a particular post has received; Leventhal, "How removing 'likes' from Instagram could affect our mental health."
91. @manicpixiememequeen, "i'll be posting sun sign moodboards over the next few days," Instagram post, March 13, 2017, accessed June 22, 2022, https://www.instagram.com/p/BRjx_shFMuD/; Julia Hava (@binchcity), "Thanks for all your submissions. Luckily this series has no end in sight because men just keep on saying dumb shit," Instagram post, May 16, 2018, accessed June 22, 2022, https://www.instagram.com/p/Bi0Qou4HKio/; Prozac.barbie, "happy materialism season!!," Instagram post, December 23, 2017, accessed June 22, 2022, https://www.instagram.com/p/BdBwmvFF0zo/.
92. Marwick, "Instafame: Luxury selfies in the attention economy."
93. "Binch City—Home," website, last accessed March 10, 2020, no longer available, https://www.binchcity.com/.
94. Julia Hava, "Julia Hava is creating a queenly community," website, accessed June 25, 2022, https://www.patreon.com/binchcity.
95. Robertson, "Inside Patreon, the economic engine of internet culture."
96. Julia Hava (@binchcity), "remember to smash your mf medication today everyone," Instagram post, July 27, 2018, accessed June 22, 2022, https://www.instagram.com/p/BltivEhHdym/.
97. Blackman, "Affective politics, debility and hearing voices."
98. Young, "How to increase serotonin in the human brain without drugs."
99. Pai, "18 New Beauty Slang Words You Need to Know."
100. Julia Hava (@binchcity), "Hi Lovelies! This is my ~Medication Haul~ Should I make more videos?," Instagram post, March 2, 2017, accessed June 22, 2022, https://www.instagram.com/p/BRJU8CHh44X/.
101. Martin et al, "Individual differences in uses of humor and their relation to psychological well-being."
102. Ibid.
103. Haley had 59,000 followers in late 2018, and toward the end of 2021, she had 110,000 followers. In December 2021, however, her account was disabled for unknown reasons and she started a backup account titled @ghosted_1996, Haley Byam (@ghosted_1996), "someone please tell me what to do," Instagram post, December 8, 2021, accessed June 27, 2022, https://www.instagram.com/p/CXO6K-TPJU6/?hl=en.

104. Haley Byam (@ghosted1996), "An old hardcore mood," Instagram post, https://www.instagram.com/p/BUq1z_lFVi9/, the post is no longer available at this link because Haley's account was suspended by Instagram and since late 2021 she has a new one under the slightly different username @ghosted_1996, see note 102.

105. Ibid.

106. Haley Byam (@ghosted1996), "Um this had a typo so reposting lol I hate myself but Raise your hand if mental healthcare/pharma has actually drastically worsened your illness but you're still dependent on it," Instagram post, https://www.instagram.com/p/BVvCOzolI5i/, just as with the post referenced in note 102, this post is no longer available.

107. Greengross, "The Relationship Between Humor and Depression;" Kfrerer, Martin and Schermer, "A behavior genetic analysis of the relationship between humor styles and depression."

108. Paper Magazine, "PAPER Predictions: 100 People Taking Off in 2019."

109. Rentschler and Thrift, "Doing feminism in the network."

110. Lawrence and Ringrose, "@Notofeminism, #Feministsareugly, and Misandry Memes," 218.

111. Ibid, 218.

112. Kanai, "Sociality and Classification: Reading Gender, Race, and Class in a Humorous Meme," 4.

113. Ibid, 4.

114. @manicpixiememequeen, "sad socialist memes," Instagram post, April 22, 2017, accessed June 22, 2022, https://www.instagram.com/p/BTMnBoGF3QS/.

115. Prozac.barbie, "happy materialism season!!," Instagram post, December 23, 2017, accessed June 22, 2022, https://www.instagram.com/p/BdBwmvFF0zo/.

116. Lawrence and Ringrose, "@Notofeminism, #Feministsareugly, and Misandry Memes," 218.

117. Ibid, 218.

118. Elyse Fox, "Conversations with Friends," Vimeo video, accessed June 25, 2022, https://vimeo.com/196129642; Jacoby, "How Instagram's 'Sad Girls Club' Is Busting the Stigma Around Mental Illness."

119. Elyse Fox (@elyse.fox), "What a Monday morning treat🏆 Thank you so much @instagram for spotlighting my newest initiative @sadgirlsclub," Instagram post, last accessed July 7, 2020, has since been deleted, https://www.instagram.com/p/BT1aeusluAM/.

120. Fluker, "How Founder Of Sad Girls Club Tackles Mental Health Issues Online;" Jacoby, "How Instagram's 'Sad Girls Club' Is Busting the Stigma Around Mental Illness;" Loggins, "Instagram 'Sad Girls Club' helps young women deal with depression;" Ross, "Elyse Fox: 'I Was Labeled As The Angry Black Woman.'"

121. Jacoby, "How Instagram's 'Sad Girls Club' Is Busting the Stigma Around Mental Illness."
122. Sad Girls Club (@sadgirlsclub), "Sad Girls at @teenvogue summit 🐱 ," Instagram post, June 2, 2018, accessed June 22, 2022, https://www.instagram.com/p/Bjh4SMsHRna/.
123. Sad Girls Club (@sadgirlsclub), "Sad Girls Club is excited and honored to represent mental health awareness and self acceptance in 🐱 @olay's 🐱 #FaceAnything campaign," Instagram post, August 21, 2018, accessed June 22, 2022, https://www.instagram.com/p/Bmv-KXSlLei/; Sad Girls Club (@sadgirlsclub), "Founder @elyse.fox shares some tips about what to do when social media becomes too overwhelming for @monki's 'All the feels,'" Instagram post, October 26, 2018, accessed June 22, 2022, https://www.instagram.com/p/BpaQD7oh0tm/.
124. Fox in Jacoby, "How Instagram's 'Sad Girls Club' Is Busting the Stigma Around Mental Illness."
125. Alderton, *The aesthetics of self-harm*, 106.
126. Sad Girls Club (@sadgirlsclub), "Do you want to help a friend who's going through IT? Here are some ways you can help," Instagram post, June 6, 2017, accessed June 22, 2022, https://www.instagram.com/p/BVAoI8-FjOB/; Sad Girls Club (@sadgirlsclub), "A HUGE reason why SadGirlsClub was created was to remove the negative stigma behind discussing mental illnesses," Instagram post, March 29, 2017, accessed June 22, 2022, https://www.instagram.com/p/BSOvDUvAymu/.
127. Blackman, "Affective politics, debility and hearing voices."
128. Sad Girls Club (@sadgirlsclub), "Question: You see signs of mental struggles on your friends Instagram... wyd?," Instagram post, September 4, 2018, accessed June 22, 2022, https://www.instagram.com/p/BnT3Zi5FaJS/.
129. Koman, "How the 23-Year-Old Meme Queens Behind @MyTherapistSays Blew Up Instagram."
130. Ibid; Lola Tash and Nicole Argiris (@mytherapistsays), "Yes I'm still watching
    Netflix, don't stop and make me question my decisions. I chose you now be happy about it. (rp from @2trashybitches)," Instagram post, February 1, 2016, accessed June 27, 2022, https://www.instagram.com/p/BBOmF98HjNY/; Lola Tash and Nicole Argiris (@mytherapistsays), "If it requires pants, I don't want to go," Instagram post, February 6, 2016, accessed June 27, 2022, https://www.instagram.com/p/BBbqBGAnjAe/.
131. Mediakix.com, "How two friends created @mytherapistsays, a 2.4+ million follower Instagram meme empire," Blog post, last accessed March 27, 2020, website is no longer available.

132. Lorenz, "Michael Bloomberg's Campaign Suddenly Drops Memes Everywhere."
133. Kanai, "Girlfriendship and sameness;" Kanai, "The best friend, the boyfriend, other girls, hot guys, and creeps;" Kanai, *Gender and Relatability in Digital Culture*; Kanai, "On not taking the self seriously."
134. Kanai, "On not taking the self seriously," 60.
135. Lola Tash and Nicole Argiris (@mytherapistsays), "Forever always on the verge of a Britney 2007 meltdown (via @tindervsreality)," Instagram post, February 19, 2016, accessed June 27, 2022, https://www.instagram.com/p/BB-kGwHnjOJ/.
136. Sieben, "Britney Spears' 2007 Mental Health Crisis Is a 2017 Meme."
137. Gill and Kanai, "Mediating Neoliberal Capitalism."
138. Kanai, *Gender and Relatability in Digital Culture*.
139. At one point in my research, the My Therapist Says website contained extensive information for potential advertisers. Including a "press" heading that featured links to several articles about the account, an "advertise"-section where companies could find information on how to purchase access to the My Therapist Says audience, boasting about "2 million impressions per post," "75K engagements per image" and "200K engagements per video." The website also featured an 8-page media kit that outlined the case for working with the My Therapist Says brand, detailing their demographic and their resume of brand partners. These pages are no longer available on their website, which at the time of writing only contains some basic information about Tash and Argiris and a webshop. "My Therapist is … rebranding," website, accessed June 27, 2022, https://mytherapistsays.ca/.
140. Institute for Precarious Consciousness, "WE ARE ALL VERY ANXIOUS."
141. Ibid.
142. Ibid.
143. Haley Byam (@ghosted1996), "An old hardcore mood," Instagram post, https://www.instagram.com/p/BUq1z_1FVi9/, the post is no longer available at this link because Haley's account was suspended by Instagram and since late 2021 she has a new one under the slightly different username @ghosted_1996; Haley Byam (@ghosted1996), "Um this had a typo so reposting lol I hate myself but Raise your hand if mental healthcare/pharma has actually drastically worsened your illness but you're still dependent on it," Instagram post, https://www.instagram.com/p/BVvCOzolI5i/, just as with the other post, this post is no longer available.
144. Haley Byam (@ghosted1996), "Anyone tried nuva ring for PMDD? Drop ur experiences in the comments below," Instagram post, just as with the Byam's other posts, this has since been deleted, https://www.instagram.com/p/BmJ42ghFyYl/.

145. Institute for Precarious Consciousness, "WE ARE ALL VERY ANXIOUS."
146. Ibid.
147. Haley Byam (@ghosted_1996), "someone please tell me what to do," Instagram post, December 8, 2021, accessed June 27, 2022, https://www.instagram.com/p/CXO6K-TPJU6/?hl=en.
148. Kanai, "On not taking the self seriously," 60.

REFERENCES

Alderton, Zoe. *The Aesthetics of Self-Harm: The Visual Rhetoric of Online Self-Harm Communities.* London and New York: Routledge, 2018. https://doi.org/10.4324/9781315637853-2.
Alfonso, Fernando. "The Real Origins of Tumblr." *The Daily Dot*, May 23, 2013. https://www.dailydot.com/business/origin-tumblr-anarchaia-projectionist-david-karp/.
Barron, Benjamin. "Richard Prince, Audrey Wollen, and the Sad Girl Theory." *I-D*, November 12, 2014. https://i-d.vice.com/en_us/article/nebn3d/richard-prince-audrey-wollen-and-the-sad-girl-theory.
Berlant, Lauren. *Desire/Love.* Brooklyn, NY: Dead Letter Office, BABEL Working Group, punctum books, 2012.
Blackman, Lisa. *Hearing Voices: Embodiment and Experience.* London and New York: Free Association Books, 2001.
Blackman, Lisa. "Affective Politics, Debility and Hearing Voices: Towards a Feminist Politics of Ordinary Suffering." *Feminist Review* 111, no. 1 (2015): 25–41. https://doi.org/10.1057/fr.2015.24.
Blackman, Lisa, and Valerie Walkerdine. *Mass Hysteria: Critical Psychology and Media Studies.* Hampshire, UK & New York: Palgrave Macmillan, 2001.
Bratich, Jack. "Occupy All the Dispositifs: Memes, Media Ecologies, and Emergent Bodies Politic." *Communication and Critical/Cultural Studies* 11, no. 1 (September 23, 2013): 64–73. https://doi.org/10.1080/14791420.2013.827351.
Calderón-Douglass, Barbara. "Sad Girls y Qué Are Breaking Down Machismo with Internet Art." *Vice*, October 24, 2014. https://www.vice.com/en_us/article/nnqkqm/sad-girls-y-que-is-breaking-down-machismo-and-offering-an-alternative-to-white-feminism-456.
Cho, Alexander. "Default Publicness: Queer Youth of Color, Social Media, and Being Outed by the Machine." *New Media and Society* 20, no. 9 (2018): 3183–3200. https://doi.org/10.1177/1461444817744784.
Cvetkovich, Ann. *Depression: A Public Feeling.* Durham and London: Duke University Press, 2012.

Decaille, Nina. "Elyse Fox's 'Sad Girls Club' Challenges The Narrative About Women Of Color & Mental Health." *Bustle.Com*, May 15, 2017. https://www.bustle.com/p/elyse-foxs-sad-girls-club-challenges-the-narrative-about-women-of-color-mental-health-57601.

Devcollab. "The Reign Of The Internet Sad Girl Is Over—And That's A Good Thing." *The Establishment*, August 24, 2017. https://theestablishment.co/the-reign-of-the-internet-sad-girl-is-over-and-thats-a-good-thing-eb6316f590d9/.

Duggan, Jamie M., N. L. Heath, Stephen P. Lewis, and Alyssa L. Baxter. "An Examination of the Scope and Nature of Non-Suicidal Self-Injury Online Activities: Implications for School Mental Health Professionals." *School Mental Health* 4, no. 1 (2012): 56–67. https://doi.org/10.1007/s12310-011-9065-6.

Eden, Nellie. "Sad Girls Y Qué." *Wonderland Magazine*, March 3, 2015. https://www.wonderlandmagazine.com/2015/03/03/sad-girls-y-que/.

Eler, Alicia. "Panel This Is What Feminism 4.0 Looks Like." *Mandatory*, May 12, 2016. https://www.mandatory.com/living/987515-panel-feminism-4-0-looks-like.

Fink, Marty, and Quinn Miller. "Trans Media Moments: Tumblr, 2011-2013." *Television and New Media* 15, no. 7 (2014): 611–26. https://doi.org/10.1177/1527476413505002.

Fluker, Dominique. "How Founder Of Sad Girls Club Tackles Mental Health Issues Online." *Forbes.Com*, October 31, 2018. https://www.forbes.com/sites/dominiquefluker/2018/10/31/sadgirlsclub/.

Freud, Sigmund. "Humour." In *Collected Papers of Sigmund Freud (Vol 5)*, edited by James Strachey. New York: Basic Books, 1959.

Freud, Sigmund. *Jokes and Their Relation to the Unconscious.* New York: Norton, 1960.

Gibbs, Anna. "Apparently Unrelated: Affective Resonance, Concatenation and Traumatic Circuitry in the Terrain of the Everyday." In *Traumatic Affect*, edited by Meera Atkinson and M Richardson, 129–47. U.K.: Cambridge Scholars Publishing, 2013.

Gill, Rosalind, and Akane Kanai. "Mediating Neoliberal Capitalism: Affect, Subjectivity and Inequality." *Journal of Communication* 68, no. 2 (2018): 318–26. https://doi.org/10.1093/joc/jqy002.

Gill, Rosalind, and Shani Orgad. "The Confidence Cult(Ure)." *Australian Feminist Studies* 30, no. 86 (2015): 324–44.

Gonzalez, Mira, and Audrey Wollen. "In Conversation with Mira Gonzalez." *Believer Magazine*, February 1, 2018. https://believermag.com/in-conversation-with-mira-gonzalez/.

Gray, Briahna Joy. "The Question of Cultural Appropriation." *Current Affairs*, September 6, 2017. https://www.currentaffairs.org/2017/09/the-question-of-cultural-appropriation.

Greengross, Gil. "The Relationship Between Humor and Depression." *Psychology Today*, November 22, 2019. https://www.psychologytoday.com/us/blog/humor-sapiens/201911/the-relationship-between-humor-and-depression.

Hines, Alice. "A Taxonomy of the Sad Girl." *I-D*, June 17, 2015. https://i-d.vice.com/en_us/article/pabzay/a-taxonomy-of-the-sad-girl.

Hochschild, Arlie Russell. *The Managed Heart: Commercialization of Human Feeling*. Berkeley, Los Angeles, London: University of California Press, 1983.

Holowka, Eileen Mary. "Between Artifice and Emotion: The 'Sad Girls' of Instagram." In *Leadership, Popular Culture and Social Change*, edited by Kristin M. S. Bezio and Kimberly Yost. Cheltenham, UK and Northampton, MA, USA: Edward Elgar Publishing, 2018.

Institute for Precarious Consciousness. "WE ARE ALL VERY ANXIOUS: Six Theses on Anxiety and Why It Is Effectively Preventing Militancy, and One Possible Strategy for Overcoming It." *Weareplanc.Org*, April 4, 2014. https://www.weareplanc.org/blog/we-are-all-very-anxious/.

Jacoby, Sarah. "How Instagram's 'Sad Girls Club' Is Busting the Stigma Around Mental Illness." *Self.Com*, October 13, 2017. https://www.self.com/story/instagram-sad-girls-club-is-busting-the-stigma-around-mental-illness.

Jadayel, Rola, Karim Medlej, and Jinan Jennifer Jadayel. "Mental Disorders: A Glamorous Attraction on Social Media?" *Journal of Teaching and Education 7*, no. 1 (2017): 465–76.

Jennings, Rebecca. "Wearing Your Emotions on Your Sleeve." *Racked*, July 1, 2016. https://www.racked.com/2016/7/1/11956536/sad-girl-fashion.

Joho, Jess. "How Being Sad, Depressed, and Anxious Online Became Trendy." *Mashable.Com*, June 28, 2019. https://mashable.com/article/anxiety-depression-social-media-sad-online/?europe=true.

Jones, Daisy. "Remembering Instagram Before the Influencers." *Vice*, July 31, 2019. https://www.vice.com/en_asia/article/pajj4n/instagram-before-influencers-arvida-bystrom-audrey-woollen.

Kanai, Akane. "Sociality and Classification: Reading Gender, Race, and Class in a Humorous Meme." *Social Media and Society* 2, no. 4 (2016). https://doi.org/10.1177/2056305116672884.

Kanai, Akane. "The Best Friend, the Boyfriend, Other Girls, Hot Guys, and Creeps: The Relational Production of Self on Tumblr." *Feminist Media Studies* 17, no. 6 (2017a): 911–25. https://doi.org/10.1080/14680777.2017.1298647.

Kanai, Akane. "Girlfriendship and Sameness: Affective Belonging in a Digital Intimate Public." *Journal of Gender Studies* 26, no. 3 (2017b): 293–306. https://doi.org/10.1080/09589236.2017.1281108.

Kanai, Akane. *Gender and Relatability in Digital Culture: Managing Affect, Intimacy and Value*. Cham: Palgrave Macmillan, 2019a. https://doi.org/10.1007/978-3-319-91515-9.

Kanai, Akane. "On Not Taking the Self Seriously: Resilience, Relatability and Humour in Young Women's Tumblr Blogs." *European Journal of Cultural Studies* 22, no. 1 (2019b): 60–77. https://doi.org/10.1177/1367549417722092.

Kfrerer, Marisa L., Nicholas G. Martin, and Julie Aitken Schermer. "A Behavior Genetic Analysis of the Relationship between Humor Styles and Depression." *HUMOR* 32, no. 3 (2019): 417–31. https://doi.org/10.1515/humor-2017-0098.

Koman, Tess. "How the 23-Year-Old Meme Queens Behind @MyTherapistSays Blew Up Instagram." *Cosmopolitan.Com*, June 20, 2017. https://www.cosmopolitan.com/lifestyle/a10027576/lola-tash-nicole-argiris-mytherapistsays-blew-up-instagram/.

Lawrence, Emilie, and Jessica Ringrose. "@Notofeminism, #Feministsareugly, and Misandry Memes: How Social Media Feminist Humor Is Calling out Antifeminism." In *Emergent Feminisms: Complicating a Postfeminist Media Culture*, edited by Jessalynn Keller and Maureen E. Ryan, 211–32. New York: Routledge, 2018.

Leventhal, Jamie. "How Removing 'Likes' from Instagram Could Affect Our Mental Health." *PBS NewsHour*, November 25, 2019. https://www.pbs.org/newshour/science/how-removing-likes-from-instagram-could-affect-our-mental-health.

Loggins, Brittany. "Instagram 'Sad Girls Club' Helps Young Women Deal with Depression." *Today.Com*, August 23, 2017. https://www.today.com/health/instagram-sad-girls-club-helps-young-women-deal-depression-t115417.

Lorenz, Taylor. "Michael Bloomberg's Campaign Suddenly Drops Memes Everywhere." *New York Times*, February 13, 2020. https://www.nytimes.com/2020/02/13/style/michael-bloomberg-memes-jerry-media.html.

Martin, Rod A., and Herbert M. Lefcourt. "Sense of Humor as a Moderator of the Relation between Stressors and Moods." *Journal of Personality and Social Psychology* 45, no. 6 (1983): 1313–24. https://doi.org/10.1037/0022-3514.45.6.1313.

Martin, Rod A., Patricia Puhlik-Doris, Gwen Larsen, Jeanette Gray, and Kelly Weir. "Individual Differences in Uses of Humor and Their Relation to Psychological Well-Being: Development of the Humor Styles Questionnaire." *Journal of Research in Personality* 37 (2003): 48–75.

Marwick, Alice E. "Instafame: Luxury Selfies in the Attention Economy." *Public Culture* 27, no. 1 (2015): 137–60. https://doi.org/10.1215/08992363-2798379.

McCosker, Anthony. "Engaging Mental Health Online: Insights from Beyondblue's Forum Influencers." *New Media and Society* 20, no. 12 (2018): 4748–64. https://doi.org/10.1177/1461444818784303.

Mondalek, Alexandra. "When Did It Become Cool to Be a 'Sad Girl'?" *Yahoo Lifestyle*, March 1, 2018. https://www.yahoo.com/lifestyle/become-cool-sad-girl-200412836.html.

Montgomery, James. "@SoSadToday: Twitter's Favorite Depressive Breaks Her Silence." *Rolling Stone*, May 28, 2014. https://www.rollingstone.com/culture/culture-news/sosadtoday-twitters-secret-superstar-speaks-for-the-first-time-88437/.

Mooney, Heather. "Sad Girls and Carefree Black Girls: Affect, Race, (Dis) Possession, and Protest." *WSQ: Women's Studies Quarterly* 46, no. 3–4 (2018): 175–94. https://doi.org/10.1353/wsq.2018.0038.

Morimoto, Lori, and Louisa Stein. "Tumblr and Fandom." *Transformative Works and Cultures* 27 (June 15, 2018). https://doi.org/10.3983/twc.2018.1580.

Newell-Hanson, Alice. "2015 the Year of... Sad Girls and Sad Boys." *I-D*, December 22, 2015. https://i-d.vice.com/en_us/article/pabvk7/2015-the-year-of-sad-girls-and-sad-boys.

O'Connell, Walter E. "Freudian Humour: The Eupsychia of Everyday Life." In *Humour and Laughter: Theory, Research, and Applications*, edited by Antony J. Chapman and Hugh C. Foot, 313–30. London: Wiley, 1976.

Orgad, Shani, and Rosalind Gill. *Confidence Culture*. Durham and London: Duke University Press, 2022. https://doi.org/10.1215/9781478021834.

Pai, Deanna. "18 New Beauty Slang Words You Need to Know." *Allure*, July 1, 2016. https://www.allure.com/story/beauty-slang-words.

Pandika, Melissa. "Sad Culture Normalizes Mental Illness. But Does It Also Glamorize It?" *Mic.Com*, November 27, 2019. https://www.mic.com/p/sad-culture-normalizes-mental-illness-but-does-it-also-glamorize-it-19406893.

PaperMagazine. "PAPER Predictions: 100 People Taking Off in 2019." *Paper Magazine*, January 29, 2019. https://www.papermag.com/paper-predictions-2625149547.html.

Petrarca, Emilia. "A Memes to an End: How Feminist Meme-Makers Are Challenging Trump's America Online." *W Magazine*, November 21, 2016. https://www.wmagazine.com/story/a-memes-to-an-end-how-feminist-meme-makers-are-challenging-trumps-america-online/.

Premack, Rachel. "Tumblr's Depression Connection." *TheRinger.Com*, October 24, 2016. https://theringer.com/tumblr-communities-depression-mental-illness-anxiety-c2ca927cd305.

Renninger, B. J. "'Where I Can Be Myself... Where I Can Speak My Mind': Networked Counterpublics in a Polymedia Environment." *New Media & Society* 17, no. 9 (2015): 1513–29. https://doi.org/10.1177/1461444814530095.

Rentschler, Carrie A., and Samantha C. Thrift. "Doing Feminism in the Network: Networked Laughter and the 'Binders Full of Women' Meme." *Feminist Theory* 16, no. 3 (2015): 329–59. https://doi.org/10.1177/1464700115604136.

Robertson, Adi. "Inside Patreon, the Economic Engine of Internet Culture." *The Verge*, August 3, 2017. https://www.theverge.com/2017/8/3/16084248/patreon-profile-jack-conte-crowdfunding-art-politics-culture.

Ross, Ashley. "Elyse Fox: 'I Was Labeled As The Angry Black Woman—But I Just Had A Chemical Imbalance In My Brain.'" *WomensHealthMag.Com*, May 12, 2017. https://www.womenshealthmag.com/health/a19993208/mental-health-instagram/.

Saxelby, Ruth. "Meet Bunny Michael, The Artist Whose Tragicomic Memes Say What Everyone Is Feeling." *The Fader*, December 20, 2016. https://www.thefader.com/2016/12/20/bunny-michael-meme-interview.

Seko, Yukari, Sean A. Kidd, David Wiljer, and Kwame J. McKenzie. "On the Creative Edge: Exploring Motivations for Creating Non-Suicidal Self-Injury Content Online." *Qualitative Health Research* 25, no. 10 (2015): 1334–46. https://doi.org/10.1177/1049732315570134.

Shane-Simpson, Christina, Adriana Manago, Naomi Gaggi, and Kristen Gillespie-Lynch. "Why Do College Students Prefer Facebook, Twitter, or Instagram? Site Affordances, Tensions between Privacy and Self-Expression, and Implications for Social Capital." *Computers in Human Behavior* 86 (2018): 276–88. https://doi.org/10.1016/j.chb.2018.04.041.

Sieben, Lauren. "Britney Spears' 2007 Mental Health Crisis Is a 2017 Meme. What Does That Say About Us?" *Brit + Co*, October 10, 2017. https://www.brit.co/britney-spears-2007-crisis-is-a-2017-meme-what-does-that-say-about-us/.

Thelandersson, Fredrika. "Social Media Sad Girls and the Normalization of Sad States of Being." *Capacious: Journal for Emerging Affect Inquiry*, November 2, 2017. https://doi.org/10.22387/CAP2017.9.

Tucker, Ian, and Lewis Goodings. "Medicated Bodies: Mental Distress, Social Media and Affect." *New Media and Society* 20, no. 2 (2018): 549–63. https://doi.org/10.1177/1461444816664347.

Tunnicliffe, Ava. "Audrey Wollen On The Power of Sadness." *NYLON*, July 20, 2015. https://nylon.com/articles/audrey-wollen-sad-girl-theory.

Vozick-Levinson, Simon. "@SoSadToday Reveals Herself—And Her Existential Beach Read." *Rolling Stone*, May 19, 2015. https://www.rollingstone.com/culture/culture-features/sosadtoday-reveals-herself-and-her-existential-beach-read-60068/.

Watson, Lucy. "How Girls Are Finding Empowerment through Being Sad Online." *Dazed Digital*, November 23, 2015. https://www.dazeddigital.com/photography/article/28463/1/girls-are-finding-empowerment-through-internet-sadness.

Wells, Emily. "Audrey Wollen's Feminist Instagram World." *Artillery Magazine*, May 3, 2016. https://artillerymag.com/audrey-wollens-feminist-instagram-world/.

Whitlock, Janis L., Jane L. Powers, and John Eckenrode. "The Virtual Cutting Edge: The Internet and Adolescent Self-Injury." *Developmental Psychology* 42, no. 3 (2006): 407–17. https://doi.org/10.1037/0012-1649.42.3.407.

Young, Simon N. "How to Increase Serotonin in the Human Brain without Drugs." *Journal of Psychiatry and Neuroscience* 32, no. 6 (2007): 394–99.

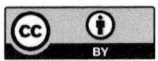

CHAPTER 6

Conclusion

In the preceding chapters I have traced how the Western media landscape of the early twenty-first century has gone from one focused on the positive to one that has room for talk about sadness and mental distress. This happened either in a way that exemplified profitable vulnerability—a marketable mental health awareness that strengthens the authenticity of celebrities and brands—or within the frames of sad girl culture—where capacious ways of feeling bad are explored and critical analyses of why we feel bad are encouraged.

In the world of magazines, this meant increased coverage of issues relating to depression, anxiety, and other diagnoses. *Cosmopolitan*'s articles on mental health largely took the same tongue-in-cheek approach as their coverage of issues like beauty, sex, and work, and did in this way place mental wellbeing into the same fold as those other everyday matters. Their earlier articles adopt an approach that assumes readers might know someone else who is struggling, and the later ones instead assume that their readers have firsthand experience of mental illness. The tone in their articles tended to take a lighthearted and distanced approach to issues of mental health, ensuring a relatable coverage that touches on difficult topics but never veers too far into uncomfortable territory.

Teen Vogue, on the other hand, often took a straightforward, earnest, and serious approach to issues of mental health, adopting the language of mental health advocacy and awareness by frequently mentioning the importance of speaking out and fighting stigma. This outlet's branding as

F. Thelandersson, *21st Century Media and Female Mental Health*,
https://doi.org/10.1007/978-3-031-16756-0_6

"woke" was reflected in the repeated connections made between mental health, inequality, and structures of oppression, as well as in their overall critical stance towards the pharmaceutical industry. Support was a key issue in *Teen Vogue*, with articles about sensitive topics frequently accompanied by the phone numbers to suicide prevention hotlines or linking to other resources. Pieces in this publication also tended to provide substantial context and information about the diagnoses and difficulties discussed, even in relation to celebrity reporting and easygoing listicles, something that was not the case in *Cosmopolitan*.

The examination of these magazines' mental health coverage shows that while *Cosmopolitan* tended to follow a script for postfeminist media— full of contradictions, covering serious topics in a tongue-in-cheek way that undermined any gravity—*Teen Vogue* offered a nuanced portrayal of mental illness that incited its readers to a more critical and engaged interpretation of the dominating biomedical paradigm. In this sense *Cosmo* exemplifies the profitable vulnerability of contemporary media culture, where difficult subjects are shared in easily digestible ways as a means to establish authenticity but ultimately feeds back into neoliberal confidence culture. *Teen Vogue's* coverage, on the other hand, was more aligned with the sad girl culture of social media, where critical approaches to feeling bad are found.

When it comes to celebrities the health narratives of Demi Lovato and Selena Gomez show that the mental breakdown and subsequent comeback narratives that were once the prerogative of male celebrities now are also available for women to adopt.[1] Lovato's repeated setbacks and confessions especially suggest that stars of all genders can now cast themselves as masters of self-transformation with the help of biomedical diagnoses and intimate confessions about what is happening behind the scenes. Gomez's health narrative confirms that acknowledgments of mental distress are available also to "spectacularized can-do" girls who were previously portrayed as always successful and well-adjusted.[2] For both Lovato and Gomez, the confessions about mental distress have served to strengthen the authenticity and realness of their celebrity brands, where their continuous struggles and the disclosure of them become the basis of intimate connections with fans. A cynical reading of their celebrity health narratives may propose that the openness about mental health is just a sign of their teams adopting to an increasingly intimate media landscape where microcelebrities have set the tone for the levels of personal details that need to be shared to maintain strong connections to fans. These aspects of their health narratives are clear examples of profitable vulnerability, where their struggles literally become valuable parts of their celebrity brands. But a more spacious analysis of what is happening would also acknowledge the support that their fans gain through them being open about these issues, as expressed by Lovato's fans in *Stay Strong* and on Twitter after the singer's 2018 overdose. In the venues and through channels about the stars, fans find each other and can get and provide support in difficult times.

In this chapter I also discuss what I term a postfeminist sadness, by accounting briefly for the emergence of Lana del Rey on the music scene in 2011–2012 and the controversy she caused at the time by displaying female weakness in a popular culture saturated with female strength. At the time del Rey was characterized as an anti-feminist for singing about female vulnerability and dependence on men, but five years later Gomez says in an interview with Vogue that she wants girls to "feel allowed to fall apart," reflecting a significant shift in dominant media culture towards female expressions of weakness.[3] The emergence of del Rey and Gomez's statement a few years later suggests that they were both responding to an overtly positive and empowerment-focused contemporary feminine culture, and that their subsequent successes speak to a yearning by audiences for representations of negative affects like sadness.

In the worlds of social media, young women write about their sadness and mental illness diagnoses in a variety of ways. For some sad girl figures (My Therapist Says) the feeling rules of neoliberalism are promoted, while others (Tumblr and Instagram sad girls, Wollen, Sad Girls Y Qué, and Sad Girls Club) explicitly contest them.

Relatability was a key theme also here, but whereas the *Cosmopolitan* coverage added humor to keep a distance from the topics, the humorous memes shared on Tumblr and Instagram often functioned as coping mechanisms that created connections between the sad girls and their followers, who could come together in their despair over the state of the world and their psyches. In this way these sad girls represent a kind of rupture in the profitable vulnerability paradigm, in that those participating in these discourses are encouraged to consider depression, anxiety, and mental illness as central aspects of life rather than something to immediately do away with. This is also why they can represent a way forward for the kind of precarity-focused consciousness raising that the *Institute for Precarious Consciousness* proposes.[4] This chapter showed that social media platforms provide several different ways of conceptualizing sadness and mental illness, from the sad girls of Tumblr who rest in the inertia of depression and romanticize the melancholy of artists like Lana del Rey, to the sad girls of Instagram who place their own struggles alongside critical readings of contemporary capitalism.

So why does it matter that more media attention was given to women undergoing depression, anxiety, and other mental illnesses? It matters because women's media culture up until this point was highly focused on the upbeat and the positive, with a tendency to privilege feelings like confidence, empowerment, shamelessness, and resilience.[5] As other scholars of the negative affects that do appear in this landscape have shown, the presence of affective dissonances may be interpreted as a problematization of the "accessibility and appeal of highly individualist career-oriented lifestyles idealised in cultural mythologies of powerful "can-do" girls."[6] But in other instances female rage enters the mediated public sphere only to be "simultaneously contained and disavowed."[7] And in yet another figuration, the repeated use of "fuck" might signal an irreverent feminist rage that rejects respectability politics along the lines of gender, race, class, and sexuality, in an ultimately hopeful way.[8]

The increased mental illness awareness that I have examined in this book functions in similar ways. Some of the attention given to women's sadness and mental illness speaks to the failure of an overtly positive women's media culture, like Audrey Wollen, Lana del Rey, and the sad girls on Instagram and Tumblr. But in other instances, like in *Cosmopolitan*, depression and anxiety are presented in relatable and distanced ways that serve to make it manageable and nonthreatening to the status quo. I contend that the increased attention to mental illness and sadness was a response to a culture overtly focused on the positive and upbeat, and that the surge in representations of negative affects spoke to the dissatisfactions among women.

Anchoring the Present in History

As I hoped to show in Chap. 2, mental illness diagnoses are neither completely discursive (socially and linguistically constructed) nor fixed neurological truths (biological facts of life that always look the same), but emerge and take shape in a complex interplay between sociocultural discourses and an ever-developing medical science. Throughout the history of Western psychology and psychiatry, the prevalence of certain diagnoses has been tied to contemporary conventions around things like gender. Hysteria, for example, was associated with the very fact of being a woman in the nineteenth century.[9] In the middle of the twentieth century, schizophrenia was commonly used as a diagnosis for unruly female behavior.[10] The latter half of the twentieth century was dominated by deinstitutionalization and the increased availability of psychopharmaceuticals. And as Jonathan Michel Metzl has argued, the introduction of a biomedical paradigm in psychiatry did not replace old psychoanalytic ideas about gender with "objective" biological understandings of the psyche.[11] Throughout the development of psychopharmacology, the connection between femininity and mental dis-ease remained strong. The "'emotional' problems [that] could be cured simply by visiting a doctor, obtaining a prescription, and taking a pill" were primarily marketed as cures against female ailments, such as "a woman's frigidity, to a bride's uncertainty, to a wife's infidelity."[12] Metzl suggests that the anxieties surrounding mothers, and the accompanying framing of psychotropic drugs as the "saviors" of women who risked to reject traditional gender roles, was in reality a worry about the destabilization of traditional family norms. As the worries about traditions changed, so did the model patient for psychopharmaceuticals. In the 1950s it was the frigid or cheating wife who needed to be medicated, in the 1960s and 1970s it was the feminist who dared to question patriarchal institutions like marriage and essentialist male-female roles. In the 1990s and early 2000s the workplace became the primary site for gender "struggles." Drugs like Prozac promised to keep the working woman cheery and optimistic so that she could perform the tasks required by her particular line of work.[13]

At the start of the twenty-first century, women's media culture was dominated by positive and upbeat messages about working hard to succeed in the workplace, so much so that women were configured as the ideal neoliberal subjects who, by enough work on the self, could reach almost infinite levels of achievement.[14] Antidepressant drugs like Prozac were used by a high number of women, but they were not widely discussed in women's media up until the mid-2010s. When they start to be discussed, alongside other experiences of living with mental illness, it is often framed as a brave choice by those speaking out, juxtaposed against a culture that tends to value only female strength. Selena Gomez's statement that girls "need to feel allowed to fall apart" is an example of this that almost holds out the promise of a culture that does not value work and success as the most important aspects of life. The onslaught of confessions by celebrities from 2015 and onwards about living with various diagnoses and traumas could in an optimistic reading be seen as "proof" that the demands of late-stage capitalism and the precarity of life in neoliberal states was finally being acknowledged as unsustainable. But many of these narratives were quickly reabsorbed in the confidence culture and rather than destabilize neoliberal ideals they worked to affirm them by modeling ways of constantly working on the self to better and optimize it. The increasingly precarious state of life in the West demands that subjects take increased responsibility for their own wellbeing and survival. Rather than challenge this notion and call for collective solutions to structural problems, the profitable vulnerability we see in celebrity health narratives and the most mainstream mental health discourses reinforce it by celebrating individualized answers to illness/difficulty.

Through Demi Lovato's health narrative, for example, we learn that pain and struggle are part of everyday life. But rather than pausing for too long to dwell on what is hurting, one should work hard to overcome difficulties and show resilience. The sequence in their second tell-all documentary, *Simply Complicated*, where life coach Mike Bayer describes how Lovato was living in a sober home without their own cellphone while working as a judge on X-factor is a telling example of this. In this figuration Lovato's main function is as a value-producing artist brand, not a human being. Not even when one is recovering from addiction (as well as dealing with bipolar disorder and bulimia) can work be put on pause. One might counter this reasoning by saying that of course Lovato has to work, they are a pop star and a multimillion business, and anything else would be out of the ordinary. And that is absolutely true, but alongside that fact is the increasingly intimate state of contemporary media. Lovato's health narrative is not presented as that of a distant and unreachable star living an extraordinary life of luxury (even if this might be the case), but is framed as ordinary and accessible to audiences through the documentaries and the star's social media accounts. Like this the singer's handling of her troubles (addiction, bipolar disorder, bulimia) is presented not as exceptional in the sense that it is only available to the rich and famous, but as common and relatable tools for self-improvement that can also be employed by their audiences. In other words, in an increasingly intimate media landscape, mental illnesses and other difficulties are acknowledged to show authenticity and build stronger connections with fans and followers, but they then tend to be configured within narratives of self-optimization and improvement so that the overcoming of tragedy gives added cadence to messages of resilience.

If the increased attention given to mental illness and sadness was an indirect response to a culture overtly focused on the positive, the way vulnerability is employed as a tool for profitability and more work on the self can be seen as one way in which neoliberal capitalism has co-opted and absorbed its own critique. By placing the causes and solutions to mental illness in a purely biomedical paradigm any sociocultural reasons for feeling bad can be ignored, and the status quo can be maintained. But I hope to have shown, throughout this book, that there also exists more spacious discourses around mental health, in both mainstream media and in the niche worlds of social media.

RELATABILITY'S POLITICAL DIMENSION AS A SOURCE OF SUPPORT AND SOLIDARITY

Beyond a cynical analysis that reads every celebrity confession as a marketing strategy, it also has to be acknowledged that the openness of celebrities and mainstream popular media provides opportunities for support to be given to fans, readers, and followers. This happens partly in the act of reading/hearing/seeing about someone with the same issues as oneself and learning that one is not alone, which may in itself serve a soothing and supportive function. But also in the possibility to connect with peers or professionals. This connection can happen between fans, like among Lovato's fans on Twitter after their overdose, between followers on social media who find each other in the comments section, or in *Teen Vogue*'s direct provision of National Suicide Prevention Hotline numbers and other resources. In all of these instances an added step, beyond merely relating to each other in recognition, happens in that some form of action occurs to better the situation for the one suffering who has sought out these media.

Relatability also has a political dimension as a source of solidarity. This is seen in *Teen Vogue*'s coverage that showed what it looks like to place usually personal and apolitical issues like mental illness in dialogue with structural issues like racism, classism, homophobia, and transphobia. By placing the emphasis on support, the magazine also showed what it looks like to provide readers with resources for tangible ways to get better. Among the sad girls on Instagram, memes that combine mental illness symptoms and political critique function to both create humor and distance from a difficult experience (living with depression/anxiety/bipolar disorder) and produce connections around the despair of the state of the world. The smooth and acritical relatability is somewhat ruptured, in that it is mixed with anticapitalist messages about things like the connections between the US health care system and Wall Street. Here users come together in humor and provide support in a critical context.

In the worlds of social media, the various iterations of the sad girl and the contexts formed there show how people can share their experiences of depression and anxiety in ways that complicate the regular biomedical narratives and function as nodes of support for those who are suffering. As discussed in the fifth chapter, this could constitute what the *Institute for Precarious Consciousness* calls a "precarity-focused consciousness raising," but it can also be another iteration of what Anne Allison calls "affective activism."[15] Allison identifies this in youth-led activism in Japan, where participants shared their own experiences of attempted suicide in an attempt to combat the high suicide rates in the country. She describes this activism as one that crafts "new forms of sociality to the end not of capital or the market … but of helping anyone/everyone survive."[16] Allison calls this "a vitalist politics that creates forms of connectedness that, quite literally, sustain people in their everyday lives."[17] The online spaces where various sad girls can express themselves and come together in their despair might be seen in a similar way. Through humorous memes immediate relief is had, users feel less alone, and support can be found.

FINAL THOUGHTS

As I am finishing this book in the summer of 2022, the world seems to have been on fire for a while. The COVID-19 pandemic is not yet over, there is a war raging in Ukraine, inflation has made the everyday costs of living increase for people all over the world, and in the US Roe vs. Wade was just overturned, making abortion illegal and setting back women's rights significantly. And that is not even mentioning the climate crisis that is already in full swing and only about to get worse, with little government action being taken to stop it. Many things, not least the future of Western liberal democracies, seem to be uncertain. In these times of upheaval, many people seem to be suffering psychologically. The World Health Organization has reported that the pandemic led to a 25% increase in the prevalence of depression and anxiety worldwide and calls on all countries to expand mental health services and support.[18]

What is clear is that media play a significant role in how people understand and take care of their mental wellbeing in this fast-changing world. During the first year of the pandemic, people in lockdown turned to friends and celebrities on social media to get support, with the spring of 2020 seeing a surge in online activity among both regular people and celebrities. If difficult subjects were approached in a relatable way so as to not become too overwhelming even in a pre-pandemic world, the same mechanism can be seen in the post-COVID media landscape. Online humorous memes about quarantine, lockdown, and mask-wearing proliferated, and the relatable approach became a way to talk about difficult things with a distance that made them less frightening and more manageable.

Since the start of the pandemic, in the world of social media multiple accounts that provide both humorous memes and tangible support have proliferated. Examples of this include Margeaux Feldman, who through the Instagram account softcore_trauma shares memes about recovering from trauma.[19] Their memes employ the language of attachment theory and polyvagal trauma therapy and clearly serve both a comedic and supportive function. On the Instagram account of writer-activist Adrienne Maree Brown supportive memes are mixed with poetry and calls to political action.[20] And Sonalee Rashatwar, who posts under the handle thefatsextherapist, is only one of many mental health professionals who share advice and support to their large group of followers.[21]

I hope that my arguments in this book have shown the role of both popular media and social media in shaping perceptions about mental health. The sites I have examined show that there are a multitude of ways to talk about mental illness and to provide support for those who are suffering. Media as sites for understanding and dealing with mental health thus need to be studied further, and taken into account in efforts to improve mental health care, not only for young girls and women, but for everyone.

NOTES

1. As I argued in the fourth chapter, the fact that Lovato came out as nonbinary in 2021 and said they use the pronouns they/them does not take away from the fact that the singer was a central figure in early twenty-first-century girl culture.
2. Projansky, *Spectacular Girls*.

3. Vogue.com, "Selena Gomez Gets Real About Anxiety."
4. Institute for Precarious Consciousness, "WE ARE ALL VERY ANXIOUS."
5. Banet-Weiser, *Empowered*; Dobson, *Postfeminist Digital Cultures*; Kanai, "On not taking the self seriously;" Orgad and Gill, *Confidence Culture.*
6. Dobson and Kanai, "From "can-do" girls to insecure and angry," 1.
7. Orgad and Gill, "Safety valves for mediated female rage in the #MeToo era," 596.
8. Wood, "Fuck the patriarchy."
9. Showalter, *The female malady.*
10. Appignanesi, *Sad, mad and bad.*
11. Metzl, *Prozac on the couch.*
12. Ibid, 72.
13. Ibid, 15.
14. Gill, "Postfeminist media culture;" Gill, "Culture and Subjectivity in Neoliberal and Postfeminist Times;" McRobbie, *The aftermath of feminism*; Ringrose and Walkerdine, "Regulating The Abject;" Scharff, "Gender and neoliberalism." See also Chap. 1 for a more elaborate discussion of this.
15. Allison, "The Cool Brand, Affective Activism and Japanese Youth;" Allison, *Precarious Japan*; Institute for Precarious Consciousness, "WE ARE ALL VERY ANXIOUS."
16. Allison, "The Cool Brand, Affective Activism and Japanese Youth," 106.
17. Ibid, 106.
18. WHO. "COVID-19 Pandemic Triggers 25% Increase in Prevalence of Anxiety and Depression Worldwide."
19. Feldman (@softcore_trauma), "Softcore_trauma," Instagram profile, accessed June 30, 2022, https://www.instagram.com/softcore_trauma/.
20. Brown (@adriennemareebrown), "Adrienne Maree Brown," Instagram profile, accessed June 30, 2022, https://www.instagram.com/adriennemareebrown/.
21. Sonalee (@thefatsextherapist), "The Fat Sex Therapist," Instagram profile, accessed June 30, 2022, https://www.instagram.com/thefatsextherapist/.

REFERENCES

Allison, Anne. "The Cool Brand, Affective Activism and Japanese Youth." *Theory, Culture & Society* 26, no. 2–3 (2009): 89–111. https://doi.org/10.1177/0263276409103118.
Allison, Anne. *Precarious Japan.* Durham and London: Duke University Press, 2013.

Appignanesi, Lisa. *Sad, Mad and Bad: Women and the Mind Doctors from 1800.* London: Virago Press, 2008.

Banet-Weiser, Sarah. *Empowered: Popular Feminism and Popular Misogyny.* Durham and London: Duke University Press, 2018.

Dobson, Amy Shields. *Postfeminist Digital Cultures: Femininity, Social Media, and Self-Representation.* New York: Palgrave Macmillan, 2015.

Dobson, Amy Shields, and Akane Kanai. "From 'Can-Do' Girls to Insecure and Angry: Affective Dissonances in Young Women's Post-Recessional Media." *Feminist Media Studies,* 2018, 1–16. https://doi.org/10.1080/1468077 7.2018.1546206.

Gill, Rosalind. "Postfeminist Media Culture: Elements of a Sensibility." *European Journal of Cultural Studies* 10, no. 2 (May 1, 2007): 147–66. https://doi. org/10.1177/1367549407075898.

Gill, Rosalind. "Culture and Subjectivity in Neoliberal and Postfeminist Times." *Subjectivity* 25 (2008): 432–45. https://doi.org/10.1057/sub.2008.28.

Institute for Precarious Consciousness. "WE ARE ALL VERY ANXIOUS: Six Theses on Anxiety and Why It Is Effectively Preventing Militancy, and One Possible Strategy for Overcoming It." *Weareplanc.Org,* April 4, 2014. https:// www.weareplanc.org/blog/we-are-all-very-anxious/.

Kanai, Akane. "On Not Taking the Self Seriously: Resilience, Relatability and Humour in Young Women's Tumblr Blogs." *European Journal of Cultural Studies* 22, no. 1 (2019): 60–77. https://doi.org/10.1177/ 1367549417722092.

McRobbie, Angela. *The Aftermath of Feminism: Gender, Culture and Social Change.* London, Thousand Oaks, New Delhi and Singapore: SAGE, 2009.

Metzl, Jonathan. *Prozac on the Couch: Prescribing Gender in the Era of Wonder Drugs.* Durham and London: Duke University Press, 2003.

Orgad, Shani, and Rosalind Gill. "Safety Valves for Mediated Female Rage in the #MeToo Era." *Feminist Media Studies* 19, no. 4 (2019): 596–603. https:// doi.org/10.1080/14680777.2019.1609198.

Orgad, Shani, and Rosalind Gill. *Confidence Culture.* Durham and London: Duke University Press, 2022. https://doi.org/10.1215/9781478021834.

Projansky, Sarah. *Spectacular Girls: Media Fascination and Celebrity Culture.* New York & London: New York University Press, 2014.

Ringrose, Jessica, and Valerie Walkerdine. "Regulating The Abject: The TV Make-over as Site of Neo-Liberal Reinvention toward Bourgeois Femininity." *Feminist Media Studies* 8, no. 3 (2008): 227–46. https://doi. org/10.1080/14680770802217279.

Scharff, Christina. "Gender and Neoliberalism: Young Women as Ideal Neoliberal Subjects." In *The Handbook of Neoliberalism,* edited by Simon Spring, Kean Birch, and Julie MacLeavy, 217–26. London: Routledge, 2016.

Showalter, Elaine. *The Female Malady: Women, Madness, and English Culture, 1830-1980.* New York: Pantheon Books, 1985.

Vogue.com. "Selena Gomez Gets Real About Anxiety—And How Therapy Changed Everything." *Vogue.Com*, March 16, 2017. https://www.vogue.com/article/selena-gomez-rehab-therapy-mental-health-depression.

WHO. "COVID-19 Pandemic Triggers 25% Increase in Prevalence of Anxiety and Depression Worldwide." Who.int, March 2, 2022. https://www.who.int/news/item/02-03-2022-covid-19-pandemic-triggers-25-increase-in-prevalence-of-anxiety-and-depression-worldwide.

Wood, Helen. "Fuck the Patriarchy: Towards an Intersectional Politics of Irreverent Rage." *Feminist Media Studies* 19, no. 4 (2019): 609–15. https://doi.org/10.1080/14680777.2019.1609232.

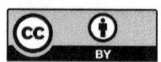

INDEX[1]

---

[1] Note: Page numbers followed by 'n' refer to notes.

© The Author(s) 2023
F. Thelandersson, *21st Century Media and Female Mental Health*,
https://doi.org/10.1007/978-3-031-16756-0